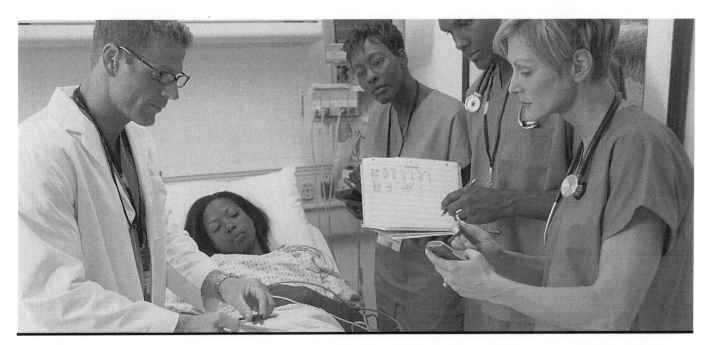

Improving Communication During Transitions of Care

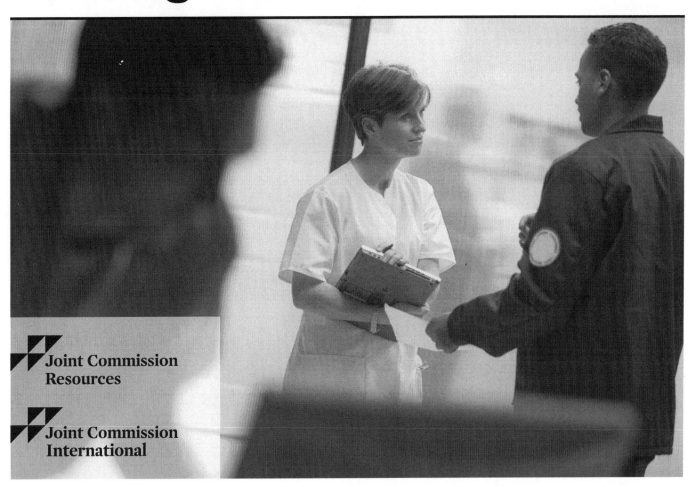

Joint Commission
Resources

Joint Commission
International

Senior Editor: Lori Meek Schuldt
Project Manager: Andrew Bernotas
Manager, Publications: Paul Reis
Associate Director, Production: Johanna Harris
Executive Director: Catherine Chopp Hinckley, Ph.D.
Joint Commission/Joint Commission International/Joint Commission Resources Reviewers: Patricia Adamski, Mary Brockway, Nanne Finis, Diane Flynn, Paul vanOstenberg

Joint Commission Resources Mission

The mission of Joint Commission Resources (JCR) is to continuously improve the safety and quality of care in the United States and in the international community through the provision of education and consultation services and international accreditation.

Joint Commission International

A division of Joint Commission Resources, Inc.

The mission of Joint Commission International (JCI) is to improve the safety and quality of care in the international community through the provision of education, publications, consultation, and evaluation services.

Joint Commission Resources educational programs and publications support, but are separate from, the accreditation activities of Joint Commission International. Attendees at Joint Commission Resources educational programs and purchasers of Joint Commission Resources publications receive no special consideration or treatment in, or confidential information about, the accreditation process.

The inclusion of an organization name, product, or service in a Joint Commission Resources publication should not be construed as an endorsement of such organization, product, or service, nor is failure to include an organization name, product, or service to be construed as disapproval.

Printed in the U.S.A. 5 4 3 2 1

Requests for permission to make copies of any part of this work should be mailed to
Permissions Editor
Department of Publications
Joint Commission Resources
One Renaissance Boulevard
Oakbrook Terrace, Illinois 60181 U.S.A.
permissions@jcrinc.com

ISBN: 978-1-59940-409-7
Library of Congress Control Number: 2010931719

For more information about Joint Commission Resources, please visit http://www.jcrinc.com.
For more information about Joint Commission International, please visit http://www.jointcommissioninternational.org.

Contents

Chapter 5: Communication in Specific Situations **71**

Chapter 6: Monitoring and Evaluating Transitions of Care **117**

Chapter 7: Case Studies on Transitions of Care **127**

Index **153**

Introduction

Consider the following scenario. A patient arrives at a hospital emergency department complaining of chest pain. A health care provider determines that the patient has suffered a mild heart attack. During the medication reconciliation process, a health care professional asks the patient about home medications but does not specifically ask about over-the-counter (nonprescription) medications, and the patient does not mention taking aspirin four times a day for arthritis pain. The patient is subsequently treated and released from the hospital with a prescription for the blood thinner warfarin.

What is the problem here?

The combination of aspirin and warfarin would put this patient at increased risk for bleeding. If information about *all* the patient's home medications had been communicated to the prescriber, the patient could have been told to discontinue the aspirin, thus avoiding a potential adverse drug event. This example illustrates the need for clear, complete communication during a transition of care.

The National Transitions of Care Coalition defines *transitions of care* as "the movement of patients between health care locations, providers, or different levels of care within the same location as their conditions and care needs change."[1] Transitions of care are also known as *handoffs/hand-offs* or *handovers/hand-overs*. The primary objective of a transition of care is to provide accurate information about a patient's care, treatment, and services; current condition; and any recent or anticipated changes.[2]

Transitions of care may occur within organizations, between organizations, or between providers. Patients often undergo multiple transitions during a single episode of care as they are transferred between units or from one provider to another during shift changes. Breakdowns in communication can occur during any transition of care and can often lead to adverse events. According to the World Health Organization (WHO) Collaborating Centre for Patient Safety Solutions,* communication breakdown during transitions of care was the leading cause of sentinel events reported to The Joint Commission between 1995 and 2006 (*see* Online Extras box; for a description of Online Extras, *see* page ix).[3] In Australia, 11% of an estimated 25,000 to 30,000 preventable adverse events that led to permanent disability were due to communication issues.[3] These and other findings were discussed in a *Patient Safety Solution* published in May 2007 to address the topic of communication during transitions of care.[3]

Online extras

To see the World Health Organization (WHO) Collaborating Centre for Patient Safety Solutions discussion and recommendations regarding communication during transitions of care, visit http://www.jcrinc.com/HCTC10/Extras/.

The Joint Commission and Joint Commission International (JCI) emphasize the importance of having a standardized approach to communication during transitions of care through their requirements for accreditation of health care

---

* In 2005, the World Health Organization designated The Joint Commission and Joint Commission International (JCI) as the WHO Collaborating Centre for Patient Safety Solutions. As the only WHO Collaborating Centre dedicated solely to patient safety, The Joint Commission and JCI further advance the entire continuum of patient safety, including principles related to system design and redesign, product safety, safety of services, and environment of care (the physical environment), as well as offering proactive solutions for patient safety, whether based on empirical evidence, hard research, or best practices. A *sentinel event,* as defined by The Joint Commission, is an unexpected occurrence involving death or serious physical or psychological injury or the risk thereof. The phrase *or the risk thereof* includes any process variation for which a recurrence would carry a significant chance of a serious adverse outcome. As defined by Joint Commission International, a *sentinel event* is an unanticipated occurrence involving death or major permanent loss of function, and an *adverse event* is an unanticipated, undesirable, or potentially dangerous occurrence in a health care organization.

organizations (*see* Online Extras box; for a description of Online Extras, *see* page ix).

In August 2009, the newly established Joint Commission Center for Transforming Healthcare embarked on a quality improvement project focused on communication during transitions of care (called "hand-off communications" in the project). A multidisciplinary team chosen by 10 leading hospitals and health systems in the United States set out to address the issues in transitions of care by using Robust Process Improvement™ (RPI), a problem-solving methodology developed by The Joint Commission. Through the use of RPI tools, the team sought to discover specific risk points and contributing factors and then to develop and implement solutions that would improve the effectiveness of communication during transitions of care. The project was expected to continue throughout 2010, culminating in the publication of the solutions in December.[4,5] To follow the progress of the project, visit the center's Web site at http://www.centerfortransforminghealthcare.org.

Joint Commission and JCI requirements are similar but different. Consult your Joint Commission or JCI accreditation manual for the specific requirements that apply to your health care organization.

Online extras

To see Joint Commission and Joint Commission International requirements related to transitions of care, visit http://www.jcrinc.com/HCTC10/Extras/.

The Purpose of This Book

Improving Communication During Transitions of Care is designed to help organizations providing all types of health care services around the world coordinate and standardize communication during transitions across the continuum of care. The book's systematic and collaborative approach to improving communication compiles considerations based on evidence-based practices, guidelines, and strategies from organizations in the field.

A Note About Terminology

In this book, to prevent confusion and ensure consistency, the term *patient* is used throughout to represent any individual receiving care, treatment, or services within or by a health care facility. The terms *caregiver* and *provider* are used in this book in a broad sense, referring to any health care professional or facility that serves patients.

Overview of Contents

Improving Communication During Transitions of Care is divided into two parts. Part 1 outlines the challenges that caregivers face when communicating during transitions of care. Part 2 provides solutions for overcoming these challenges. It discusses initiatives that various organizations have developed to improve transitions of care and includes many examples of tools, such as forms, checklists, and procedures. A brief description of each chapter follows.

Chapter 1: Communication Challenges Between Caregivers

This chapter examines nearly a dozen types of transitions a patient may experience and the problems that can arise between personnel involved in the communication at these transition points. The discussion includes transitions within an organization and transitions between two separate care facilities.

Chapter 2: Patient Experience, Participation, and Understanding of Condition

This chapter provides information about the difficulties that patients face when trying to understand their diagnoses or conditions and to participate in their care. It includes information about inadequate discharge preparation, low health literacy, and language barriers.

Chapter 3: Medication Errors

As discussed in this chapter, medication errors often occur because the organization's medication reconciliation process is inadequate or nonexistent. Another source of medication error is improper medication administration. An additional issue that can lead to error is lack of medication adherence by patients.

Chapter 4: Tools Applicable to Communication at Any Transition Point

This chapter provides a variety of tools to help standardize transitions of care at any point of patient transfer. The tools include those developed by The Joint Commission and by other organizations, along with sample forms and checklists. The chapter also features a discussion about using technology to streamline transition-of-care processes.

Chapter 5: Communication in Specific Situations

The unique considerations of specific transition points are the focus of this chapter. It includes examples of tools useful in such specific situations as a transition between a primary care physician and a specialty care provider, between an anesthesiologist and a postanesthesia recovery room nurse, at nursing shift changes, between the emergency department and another department or unit within the hospital, and between two separate care facilities.

Chapter 6: Monitoring and Evaluating Transitions of Care

This chapter includes information about conducting a failure mode and effects analysis on transitions of care and about what to look for when monitoring transition-of-care processes. In addition, the Care Transitions Measure™ tool is introduced and explained. This tool is used to monitor the transition between hospital and home. The chapter also includes descriptions of general performance improvement methodologies recommended by the Joint Commission Center for Transforming Healthcare.

Chapter 7: Case Studies on Transitions of Care

This chapter highlights initiatives that various organizations worldwide have developed to improve their transition-of-care processes. The case studies discuss the development and implementation of these initiatives as well as how they are monitored. Forms, checklists, and other tools are provided.

Online Extras

You will find bonus features related to this book on the Joint Commission Resources Web site. These Online Extras include additional examples and supplemental information. As shown earlier in this introduction, look for the box with the **online extras** icon. The Online Extras for this book are available at http://www.jcrinc.com/HCTC10/Extras/.

Acknowledgments

We are grateful to our expert manuscript reviewers:
- Patricia Adamski, R.N., M.S., M.B.A., director, Standards Interpretation Group and The Office of Quality Monitoring, The Joint Commission
- Mary Brockway, R.N., M.S., associate director, Division of Standards and Survey Methods, The Joint Commission
- Nanne Finis, R.N., M.S., executive director, Solutions Consulting, Joint Commission Resources
- Diane Flynn, R.N., M.B.A., consultant, Joint Commission Resources

- Jorge César Martinez, M.D., director, Department of Pediatrics, Safety and Quality, Universidad del Salvador, Buenos Aires, Argentina; member, Joint Commission International Editorial Advisory Board
- Rick Morrow, Master Black Belt
- Paul vanOstenberg, D.D.S., M.S., senior executive director, International Accreditation and Standards, Joint Commission International

We greatly appreciate the additional assistance of Anne Marie Benedicto, M.P.H., M.P.P.A., chief of staff and executive vice president, Support Operations, The Joint Commission.

We also gratefully acknowledge the time and insights of the following people and organizations:
- American Academy of Family Physicians
- American College of Chest Physicians
- Boston Medical Center
- Tina Budnitz, M.P.H., senior advisor, Society of Hospital Medicine
- Eric Coleman, M.D., M.P.H.
- Carole Conrad, R.N., P.C.C.N., and Maryann Cone, C.O.O., Sharp Grossmont Hospital, La Mesa, California
- Doctors Hospital, Baptist Health South Florida
- Richard Frankel, Ph.D., research scientist, Health Services Research and Development Center on Implementing Evidence-Based Practice, Richard L. Roudebush Veterans Affairs Medical Center, Indianapolis
- Jeffrey Greenwald, M.D., S.F.H.M, Project BOOST
- Griffith University, Australia
- Hamad Medical Corporation, Doha, Qatar
- Institute for Healthcare Improvement
- Jessica M. Martin, M.S., Project RED project manager, Department of Family Medicine, Boston Medical Center
- MCGHealth, Augusta, Georgia
- Kaiser Permanente, Oakland, California
- Medical Center of Central Georgia
- Miami Valley Hospital, Dayton, Ohio
- Mount Carmel East Hospital, Columbus, Ohio
- National Patient Safety Foundation
- National Transitions of Care Coalition
- OSF St. Joseph Medical Center, Bloomington, Illinois
- Parkwest Medical Center, Knoxville, Tennessee
- Mary Ann Preskul-Ricca, M.P.P., public affairs coordinator, Massachusetts Association of Health Plans
- Louise Rabøl, M.D., Copenhagen
- Jane Schetter, R.N., M.S.N., C.N.S, senior CSR consultant, Joint Commission Resources

- Vicki Alexandra Scruby, assistant executive director, Home Health Services, Hamad Medical Corporation, Doha, Qatar
- Efrat Shadmi, Ph.D., R.N., Cheryl Spencer Department of Nursing, Faculty of Social Welfare and Health Sciences at Haifa University, Israel
- Divya Shroff, M.D., associate chief of staff, Informatics, Veterans Affairs Medical Center, Washington, D.C.
- Helen Siegel, R.N., M.S., M.B.A., director of regulatory and clinical affairs, Home Health Care Association of Massachusetts
- Darrell Solet, M.D., cardiology fellow, University of Texas, Southwestern Medical Center, Dallas

- Joan Spicer, R.N., Ph.D., director, University of California San Francisco Medical Center Case Management/Social Work/Home Health Care
- University of California, Irvine
- U.S. Pharmacopeia
- WakeMed Health & Hospitals, Raleigh, North Carolina
- Mark V. Williams, M.D., F.A.C.P., F.H.M., professor and chief, Division of Hospital Medicine, Northwestern University Feinberg School of Medicine, Chicago

We also appreciate the contributions of writer Julie Henry, R.N., and the additional assistance of writers Meghan Pillow, R.N., and Felicia Schneiderhan.

References

1. National Transitions of Care Coalition: *Transitions of Care Measures*. 2008. http://www.ntocc.org/portals/0/ TransitionsOfCare_Measures.pdf (accessed Jul. 27, 2010).

2. The Joint Commission: *Comprehensive Accreditation Manual for Hospitals: The Official Handbook*. Oak Brook, IL: Joint Commission Resources, 2010.

3. WHO Collaborating Centre for Patient Safety Solutions: Communication during patient hand-overs. *Patient Safety Solutions* 1, May 2007. http://www.ccforpatientsafety.org/common/ pdfs/fpdf/presskit/PS-Solution3.pdf (accessed Jul. 27, 2010).

4. Joint Commission Center for Transforming Healthcare: *Facts About Hand-Off Communications*. http://www.centerfortransforminghealthcare.org/projects/ about_handoff_communication.aspx (accessed Jul. 27, 2010).

5. Joint Commission Center for Transforming Healthcare: *About the Center*. http://www.centerfortransforminghealthcare.org/ about/about.aspx (accessed Jul. 27, 2010).

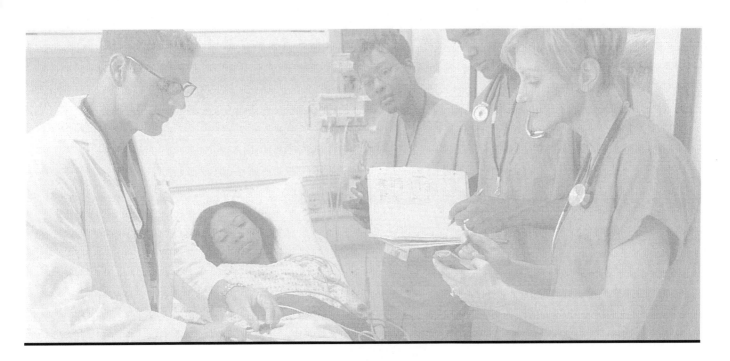

Part 1

Issues in Transitions of Care

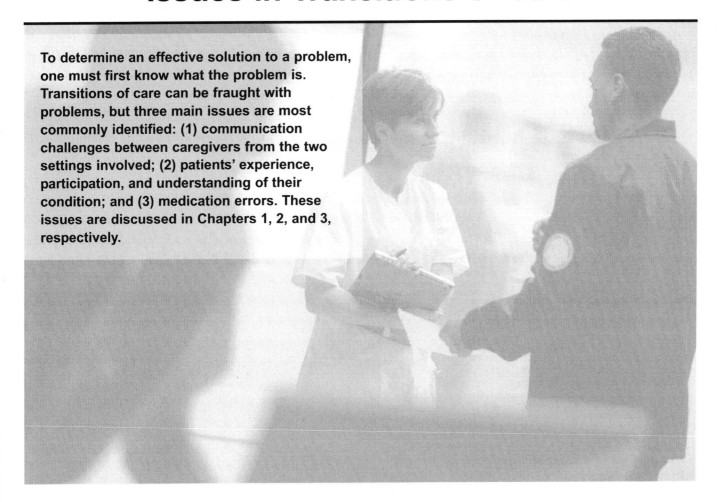

To determine an effective solution to a problem, one must first know what the problem is. Transitions of care can be fraught with problems, but three main issues are most commonly identified: (1) communication challenges between caregivers from the two settings involved; (2) patients' experience, participation, and understanding of their condition; and (3) medication errors. These issues are discussed in Chapters 1, 2, and 3, respectively.

Chapter 1

Communication Challenges Between Caregivers

Lack of complete, accurate communication between the giver and the receiver of patient information at points of transition is a major issue affecting the quality and safety of patient care. This chapter includes a discussion of challenges faced during some of the most common types of transitions of care. Solutions that address these challenges are discussed in Chapter 5.

Between Primary Care Physicians and Other Physician Specialties

Information sharing between primary care physicians and other physicians can help preserve continuity of care and limit duplication of tests and treatments.[1,2] Studies show that there are benefits to continuity of care, including fewer calls for emergency and hospital services, greater use of preventive care measures, reduction in disease-specific symptoms, and improved patient satisfaction.[1] Conversely, lack of information sharing between primary care physicians and other physician specialists has been shown to have an adverse effect on patient care.[2]

In a follow-up study of patients who were discharged from 11 Canadian hospitals in five cities, it was found that physicians received information from the patient's previous visit with another physician in only 22% of their patient visits.[1] In another study conducted in the United States, almost 10% of physicians said that they never received a case report from a referring physician, about 12% said they never received an x-ray or x-ray report, about 9% reported never receiving clinical records other than x-rays, and almost 2% said they never received a reason for referral.[2]

Communication between primary care physicians and other physician specialties can be challenging for many reasons, including the following:
- Lack of technology to generate reports easily
- Patient not disclosing visits to another physician

- Failure to request information due to perceived irrelevance to the patient's current problem
- No clearly defined referral or consultation process
- Time required for adequate communication

Between Primary Care Physicians and Hospital-Based Caregivers

High-quality patient care is dependent on good communication between primary care physicians and hospital-based caregivers. However, studies show a deficit in the quality of communication when patients make a transition from one provider to another.[3]

Continuity of care depends on provider awareness of the patient's condition, patient use of preventive services, follow-up visits, diagnosis and management of conditions, and collaboration between health care providers.[4] Communication deficiencies between physician's offices and acute care facilities contribute to the breakdown of continuity of care.[4]

In Norway, communication between primary care physicians and hospital-based physicians takes place through referral and discharge letters.[3] In Australia, patients are given a discharge letter to hand-deliver to their primary care provider.[5] In the United States, discharge summaries are sent directly to the primary care provider, usually via fax.

Information received by primary care providers following a patient emergency department visit or hospital discharge often lacks one or more of the following[5]:
- Diagnosis
- Clear discharge plan
- Diagnostic test results
- Laboratory results
- Medication changes

Between Hospitalists and Other Physicians or Other Service Units

Hospitalists—that is, physicians who specialize in the comprehensive medical care of hospitalized patients (*see* Sidebar 1-1)—participate in numerous transitions of care for every patient each day. Hospitalists facilitate patient transitions to and from physicians in multiple areas within and around the hospital, including the emergency department, the operating room, surgical services, intensive care units, the offices of primary care physicians, other hospitals, and other care facilities such as rehabilitation centers, nursing homes, and other short term and long term care facilities. Hospitalists also routinely transfer their patients among the members of their group, including between shifts and at the beginning and end of their blocks of service time.

Points of transition between care providers are vulnerable times for patients and can lead to harm if any break occurs in the flow of patient information. Transitions of care within the hospital are numerous, often happening several times a day. Inadequate communication during any of these transitions can lead to patient harm. In a survey of residents at one academic medical center, 59% reported that one or more of their patients had been harmed during their most recent clinical duty due to a problematic transition.[6]

Transitions out of the hospital also carry the risk of inadequate communication because the caregiver receiving the patient does not have direct access to the hospital records. A systematic review of communication between hospitalists and primary care physicians found that direct communication occurred infrequently (3%–34%) and that the availability of a discharge summary at the first visit after discharge was low (12%–34%). Lack of postdischarge information was found to affect the quality of care in approximately 25% of follow-up visits.[7]

At Physicians' Transfer of Complete or On-Call Responsibility

Inadequate communication between physicians often results in errors, many of which are preventable. According to Darrell Solet, M.D., cardiology fellow at the University of Texas Southwestern Medical Center in Dallas, Texas, the biggest contributor to poor communication between physicians is the physical setting in which transitions of care are conducted.[8] Solet says they "are often done in a noisy setting with poor lighting, which is not conducive to good

---

Sidebar 1-1. What Is a Hospitalist?

A hospitalist is a physician who specializes in the practice of hospital medicine, a medical specialty dedicated to the delivery of comprehensive medical care to hospitalized patients. Following medical school, hospitalists typically undergo residency training in general internal medicine, general pediatrics, or family practice but may also receive training in other medical disciplines.

In the United States, some hospitalists undergo additional postresidency training specifically focused on hospital medicine or acquire other indicators of expertise in the field, such as the Society of Hospital Medicine's Fellowship in Hospital Medicine (FHM) or the American Board of Internal Medicine's Recognition of Focused Practice (RFP) in Hospital Medicine.

Source: Society of Hospital Medicine: *Definition of a Hospitalist and Hospital Medicine.* Nov. 4, 2009. http://www.hospitalmedicine.org/AM/Template.cfm?Section= Hospitalist_Definition&Template=/CM/HTMLDisplay.cfm& ContentID=24835 (accessed Jul. 19, 2010).

---

interaction." He adds, "In many cases, there is no face-to-face interaction at all. If you're lucky you'll get an abbreviated summary of the patient's history and physical with an assessment and plan, but that's pretty rare. Often all you get is a list of patient names with an admitting diagnosis. The process is very inconsistent among physicians."[8]

In early 2005, Solet and several other researchers evaluated the care transition process at Indiana University School of Medicine's Internal Medicine Residency Program. At the time, Solet was a senior resident at Indiana University, and he became interested in studying resident processes for transitions of care at the university when one of his patients was nearly sent for an unnecessary procedure. Solet recalls, "The procedure was ordered by an on-call team that didn't understand the long-term plan for the patient. The only reason we caught it in time was because we arrived for rounds as the radiologist was at the bedside explaining the procedure to the patient."[8] Fellow researcher Richard Frankel, Ph.D., a research scientist for the Health Services Research and Development Center on Implementing Evidence-Based Practice at the Richard L. Roudebush Veterans Affairs Medical Center in Indianapolis, adds, "At the time, residents rotated through five different hospitals with five different sets of expectations."[8] Frankel says there was "a significant variation" in the way transitions of care were handled.[8]

Solet and Frankel conducted a national survey of medical schools to find out how many offered formal training in communication during transitions of care. "With all the national interest in medical errors, we were surprised to find that only 8% had a formal program," Frankel says.[8]

In 2005, a survey was conducted of on-call general surgery house officers in 17 hospitals in Wales.[9] Six of the 17 hospitals had no allocated place for transitions of care, and interruptions during transitions were common in all the hospitals.[9] Only 2 hospitals had a standardized form for transitions of care. Six of the house officers said they "never" received feedback about their patient care decisions; five said they "sometimes" received feedback. Eight said they "never" or "rarely" presented to the consultant on call.[9]

In a study conducted in the United Kingdom that simulated transitions of care using fictional patient scenarios, junior physicians who received verbal reports during transitions could not remember 67% of the information they were given after the first patient and forgot 97% of the information by the time they got to the fifth patient.[10] Among those who took notes during verbal transitions of care, 85.5% of important patient data was retained after the fifth patient.[10]

Between Anesthesiologists and Postanesthesia Recovery Room Nurses

Given the complexity of surgery today, patients are at an increased risk of errors, particularly if adequate information is not communicated during transitions of care. A surgical patient may be more vulnerable to errors related to poor communication because of the number of transitions he or she undergoes during a single procedure.[11]

Each area of the surgical environment requires a different type of expertise. Although anesthesiologists and postanesthesia recovery room nurses are both involved in the patient's surgical experience, they have distinct roles. Therefore, effective communication between the two is essential.[11]

Factors that can affect communication between anesthesiologists and postanesthesia recovery room nurses include the following[12]:
• Quick turnover of patients

• High volume of patients
• Performing multiple tasks simultaneously
• Frequent interruptions
• Noisy environment

At Nursing Shift Changes

Change-of-shift reporting between nurses is one of the more common care transitions in health care organizations. Because the information exchanged during a nursing shift change will be used to guide the patient's care during the next shift, it is crucial that relevant patient information be transferred from one nurse to the next.[12]

Proper communication between nurses at all points during a patient's hospital stay can be difficult due to high patient turnover, a lack of overlap between shifts, and time constraints. The increasing use of agency nurses and the large number of nurses involved in each patient's care add to this difficulty. Other reasons for gaps in information handed from one nurse to another include the following[13]:
• New admissions just prior to shift change
• Time available to conduct transitions of care
• Lack of knowledge about an individual patient's condition
• Focus on tasks performed rather than patient outcomes

Between Nurses and Physicians

Communication between nurses and physicians is often fraught with tension. In 2009, the results of a survey conducted by the American College of Physician Executives revealed that nearly 85% of the nurses and physicians who responded had experienced degrading comments and insults at their organizations. "It's the everyday lack of respect and communication that most adversely affects patient care and staff morale," noted one respondent.[14] Yet the behavior problems reported by respondents also included yelling, cursing, refusing to speak or work with someone, spreading malicious rumors, trying to get someone disciplined or fired unjustly, throwing objects, sexual harassment, and physical assault.[14]

Another study, ominously titled "Silence Kills," reported that more than 20% of health care professionals have seen patients harmed as a result of disrespectful and abusive behavior between physicians and staff members and that fewer than 7% of doctors or nurses who witness such behavior confront the person who is behaving that way.[15] Some nurses who participated in the American College of Physician Executives survey said that when they did report disruptive behavior by physicians, the people assigned to investigate the complaint—who were other physicians—did not take the nurses seriously and did not impose any penalty on the physicians who had been cited, yet nurses who were reported for disruptive behavior usually were fired.[14]

The relationship between physicians and nurses in Spain was found to be even more hierarchical than in the United States. Nurses reportedly were rarely consulted about patients, were infrequently included as participants in rounds, were unlikely to speak up with a concern, and were never invited to physician conferences.[16] As a result, communication between the two types of providers was incomplete and ineffective.

Why is communication between nurses and physicians so difficult? In part it is because nurses and physicians have different ways of communicating. Nurses tend to take a narrative approach, whereas physicians typically use a more focused approach in an attempt to determine the problem and fix it. Other factors that contribute to ineffective communication between nurses and physicians include the following:

- Differences in gender
- Differences in culture
- Multitasking
- Limitations of short-term memory
- Fatigue
- Stress
- Sleep deprivation
- Working in a fast-paced environment
- Intimidation due to the hierarchical system of health care organizations

Nurses and physicians frequently communicate through verbal reports, yet nurses receive little or no education about how to communicate with physicians or how to communicate effectively in urgent situations.[17] Most nurses who have recently graduated have minimal experience with contacting physicians to give status reports.[17] New nurses also may be intimidated by physicians, which may cause them to take a "hint and hope" approach—that is, instead of making direct, clear statements to the physician, the nurse only hints at what the situation is and hopes that the physician will detect its urgency and respond accordingly, but that often is not what happens.[18] This technique also has been noted in commercial aviation. Numerous examples of "black box" recordings found after airline crashes found that copilots were using the "hint and hope" approach even as the plane was going down.[18]

Other issues that contribute to poor communication between nurses and physicians include the following[18]:

- Lack of structured policies and procedures related to the content, timing, or purpose of verbal reports
- No shared mental model or framework for verbal health care communication
- No rules for verbal transmission of information, either face-to-face or on the telephone
- Differing opinions, even among nurses, about what information should be communicated during a verbal report
- Frequent interruptions and distractions
- Infrequent communication
- Lack of examples of respect and good communication among role models and leaders

Between the Emergency Department and Another Department or Unit Within the Hospital

Transfer of a patient from the emergency department (ED) to an inpatient unit is a complex process with great potential for error.[19,20] This transition of care can put the patient at risk because it requires changes in three domains[20]: (1) provider, (2) department, and (3) location. These changes may not necessarily occur simultaneously.[20]

ED personnel spend a great deal of time communicating— with each other, with the patient, or with clinicians outside the department. Thus, errors involving the ED often are linked to poor communication.[21]

Between Emergency Department Physicians and Internists

Communication between ED physicians and internists most often occurs verbally, either in person or by telephone.[21] Verbal communication between ED physicians and internists can be challenging for the following reasons[19,22]:

- Frequent interruptions
- "Telephone tag" (inability to reach one another directly over the phone)
- Competing demands on physicians' time
- Rapidly changing patient information
- Differences in expectations

Emergency departments can be busy places. When physicians are busy, sign-out may be rushed and not as interactive as it would be under better circumstances. It is also common for busy physicians to be unaware of new developments or current vital signs if they have not seen the patient recently prior to sign-out. If the admitting physicians are also busy, they may not have an opportunity to examine and treat patients immediately after transfer.[20]

Laboratory results also have a tendency to get overlooked during transfer of a patient from the ED physician to the internist. The receiving physician may not always be aware of the lab results, and laboratory personnel sometimes contact the wrong provider with urgent results during transition of responsibility for the patient.[20]

In some organizations, there is confusion about who is responsible for diagnosing the patient.[20,21] Internists may believe that diagnosis is the ED physician's responsibility, whereas the ED physicians believe that their responsibilities are limited to triage, stabilization, and transfer.[20]

"Boarding" of a patient in the emergency department until a bed becomes available can also lead to communication problems between the ED physician and the receiving internist. Even though ED physicians often are technically responsible for patients during boarding, in practice, when the ED physician gets busy, the boarding patient may be left in limbo, sometimes for hours at a time.[18] Sign-out typically occurs while the patient is still boarding, and the internist may not be updated on the patient's current condition until just prior to the patient's arrival on the unit.[18]

Between Emergency Department Nurses and Receiving Nurses

The transfer of information between emergency department nurses and unit nurses is critical to continuity of care. When patients are transferred to the emergency department, the receiving nurse often has no prior knowledge of the patient or the patient's condition, which makes clear and accurate sharing of information essential.[23]

The transfer of patients from the ED nurse to the unit nurse may be challenging for many reasons. In some instances, the ED nurse and the receiving nurse may have different understandings of when the transfer of responsibility for the patient actually begins. Some nurses may think it begins with the first call to the unit to inform the receiving nurse that the patient is being transferred; others may believe that the transition of care is not complete until all the essential information about the patient has been communicated directly to the receiving nurse.[23]

When they arrive on the receiving unit, ED nurses sometimes find it difficult to identify the nurse who should be receiving the patient. This identification can be particularly difficult in critical care areas, such as the intensive care unit, because the receiving nurse is busy concentrating on the patient's physical care and may not initially have time to focus on the information being shared.[23]

ED nurses and unit nurses often do not have a clear understanding of one another's roles, which makes it difficult for the ED nurse to know what information needs to be shared during a transition of care. Lack of a standardized process for transitions of care is a major contributor to this issue.[23]

Between Two Separate Care Settings

Communication between organizations during transitions of care may be one of the most difficult types of communication due to differences in organizational policies and a lack of familiarity between staff. Health care facilities often operate independently of one another, so they sometimes end up providing care without needed information from the transferring site. The transition between settings also includes the process of transport—for example, by ambulance or helicopter—from one facility to another. Poor transitions between settings can result in costly duplication of services and adverse patient outcomes.[24]

Between Hospital and Home Care

Home care services is a general term that includes but is not limited to the following:

- **Home health,** which provides nursing, therapy, aide, and social work services on a per-visit basis
- **Hospice,** which provides nursing, social work, chaplain, and volunteer services primarily in the home for patients who are considered terminally ill. However, these services may also be provided in a long term care facility, assisted living facility, or hospital
- **Infusion companies/pharmacies** that provide medications including intravenous antibiotics and total parenteral nutrition, supplies, and pumps in the home
- **Equipment companies,** which provide a variety of products and services, such as oxygen, ventilators, continuous positive airway pressure (CPAP) devices, hospital beds, and ambulatory aids
- **Private duty agencies** that provide nursing, aide, or homemaker services on an hourly basis

The Agency for Healthcare Research and Quality reports that the rate of patients needing home care after hospitalization increased 53% between 1997 and 2006.[25] Because people are living longer and being discharged from the hospital sooner, the typical hospital patient is now older and often requires more care than a hospital patient did 10 years ago.[26] Yet sometimes patients who would benefit from and qualify for home care services are not given the appropriate referral, and even in cases in which a referral to a home care service is made, communication of the referral is often done at the last minute.

According to a home health social worker, communication between hospitals and home care organizations often consists of the home health agency's asking the hospital to fax information about the patient. In the past, someone from the hospital would visit the patient's home prior to discharge. Today, environmental problems are dealt with as they arise, and many patients are sent home without the right medications or equipment. Frequently, even if they do have the right equipment, they do not know how to use it.[26]

Many patients who are being transferred from the hospital to home care arrive home with the misconception that someone will be waiting there to help them. In reality, the home health workers will not be there the majority of the time, so the patients are left to fend for themselves.[26]

Between Hospital and Long Term Care or Rehabilitation Facilities

Effective communication during transfer to long term care or rehabilitation facilities is critical to a patient's recovery. Patients who are being transferred to subacute facilities have special needs, so transfer of care can be a particularly vulnerable time for them.[27]

Some common problems related to transfer from the hospital to a subacute care facility include the following[27]:
• Test results pending at discharge
• Unexplained discrepancies between preadmission and discharge medication regimens
• Discharge summaries missing key information (for example, test results, pertinent lab results, information about treatment or hospital course, discharge medications, patient or family counseling, follow-up plans)

Between Hospital Emergency Departments and Nursing Homes

Nursing home residents are frequent visitors to the emergency department. In fact, almost 25% of all nursing

home residents visit the emergency department at least once a year, and more than 10% are seen two or more times each year.[24]

Transitions of care between the hospital and the nursing home can be challenging because the resident is cared for in five domains during one episode of emergency care[24]:
1. The nursing home before the emergency department visit
2. The ambulance on the way to the emergency department
3. The emergency department
4. The ambulance on the way back from the emergency department
5. The nursing home after the emergency department visit

More than 70% of nursing home residents have one or more of the following tests done while in the emergency department[24]:
• Blood tests
• Chest x-rays
• Electrocardiograms (EKGs)

Most nursing home residents are also given medications while in the emergency department.[24]

According to the literature, when nursing home residents are transferred to the emergency department, the ambulance drivers and the emergency department frequently receive no written report or verbal communication from the nursing home. Conversely, nursing homes report that residents often are returned to the nursing home with no copy of the ED chart and no treatment recommendations.[24]

Between Psychiatric Hospitals and Community Care Facilities

Patients with severe mental illness are at high risk for readmission due to disabling symptoms such as delusions, hallucinations, social withdrawal, and decreased motivation.[28] One of the major problems psychiatric patients have after hospital discharge is medication adherence. As many as 50% of patients with schizophrenia have failed to take their medications at some point; between 30% and 40% of patients with bipolar disorder have been found to be nonadherent at times.[28]

Because medication nonadherence can be an issue for patients with mental illnesses, it is important that accurate information about medication regimens be communicated to the community care facility. Failure to take medications can result in rehospitalization.

Within Specific Types of Nonhospital Settings

Each health care setting has its own unique challenges related to transitions of care. This section includes discussion about issues in communication during transitions of care within behavioral health care, long term care, and home care.

Behavioral Health Care

Caring for people with behavioral or mental health issues requires a certain level of knowledge. In today's world, many behavioral health care organizations increasingly must rely on agency or temporary staff due to a shortage of skilled professionals to fill open positions.[29] The agency staff members are then placed in settings with patients they do not know. To make sure that incoming staff members are well informed about the condition of each patient, care transitions are taking longer, and thus less time is left for patient care. Adding to the problem are higher acuity rates, higher occupancy rates, and the need for multidisciplinary interaction.[29]

Changing work patterns in the 2000s also have affected transitions of care in behavioral health care. There is a growing recognition that lengthy workdays can lead to staff errors. There is also greater emphasis on creating a healthy balance between work and leisure time for staff. As a result, staff work shifts have become shorter, and the number of transitions has increased.[29]

Long Term Care

In the long term care setting, the telephone is often the primary means of communication between nurses and physicians. Many calls are received after hours by covering physicians, leaving physicians to make important clinical decisions for patients they do not know using only the information they are given by the nurse over the telephone.[30] Therefore, to make sure the information being provided will result in good medical decisions, it is important to understand the perceived barriers to nurse-to-physician communication in long term care (*see* Sidebar 1-2).

Nurses face some challenges when working with physicians who are not familiar with the patients. Some nurses have encountered physicians who seemed angry that the issue was not addressed during regular business hours. According to one nurse, "The on-call doctor was very upset that I did not call before 5 o'clock, and I said to him that I will make sure I will tell my patients to bleed between the hours of 9 and 5."[30]

Home Care

When relevant information is not shared during transitions of care, patients are placed at risk for adverse events. Because home care agencies receive referrals from multiple hospitals, nursing homes, rehabilitative facilities, and physicians, they may be more likely than other types of organizations to receive incomplete information during transitions of care.[31] A discharge summary often is not enough to communicate all the necessary information, particularly early in the home care process when the home care nurse is just getting to know the patient.[32]

Home care referral information may be nonexistent or may consist only of the patient's name, address, and phone number. Sometimes the information is flawed. In other instances, critical pieces of information about the patient may be missing, such as the following:

• The presence of an open area on the patient's skin
• The fact that the patinet has a communicable disease such as methicillin-resistant *Staphylococcus aureus*
• Psychosocial information, such as the fact that the caregiver did not want to take the patient home
• The critical result of a particular test, such as protime, drug level, or oxygen saturation

---

Sidebar 1-2. Perceived Barriers to Communication Between Nurses and Physicians in Long Term Care Settings

Long term care nurses have identified the following as barriers to good nurse-to-physician communication:
• Feeling like they are being rushed
• Feeling that the physician does not want to deal with the problem
• Lack of consideration of their views
• Frequent interruptions
• Difficulty reaching the physician by telephone
• Finding adequate time to make a call
• Being interrupted by the physician during the report
• Lack of respect or rude behavior
• Difficulty understanding the physician (due to a heavy accent or to excessive medical jargon)

Source: Tjia J., et al.: Nurse-physician communication in the long-term care setting: Perceived barriers and impact on patient safety. *J Patient Saf* 5:145–152, Sep. 2009.

Home care nurses must work closely with the patient's physician because they rely on the physician for orders for the patient's care. However, many home care nurses have found that when they call the patient's physician to discuss the patient's needs, the physician was not even aware that the patient had been admitted to the hospital.[32] There is a particular problem when a hospitalist orders home care. Following up with patients after they leave the hospital is not part of a hospitalist's job, and thus a hospitalist may be unwilling to provide home care orders. And even when the hospitalist believes home care is appropriate, in many cases the hospitalist has not communicated with the patient's primary physician. Thus, when the home care service representative calls the patient's primary physician, the physician may refuse to provide home care orders because the physician was not aware the patient had been in the hospital and does not have the most up-to-date information about the patient. In such situations, the home care service and the patient are caught in the middle without a physician to perform needed services. The patient may have to be sent back to the hospital because a physician will not respond to a condition change.

Another problem that home care nurses face during transitions of care occurs when the patient has been told that the nurse will provide certain services when in fact the nurse actually will be teaching the patient how to perform self-care. For example, a patient might be told that a nurse will provide wound care when the home care nurse's role is to teach the patient how to care for the wound.[32]

Another difficult aspect of communication within home care organizations is medication reconciliation, which may require contacting multiple providers, including the patient's pharmacist. A particular problem exists with duplicative therapy because the patient does not recognize the difference between the generic name and the brand name of a particular medication. Thus, for example, a patient may resume the Lanoxin he or she was taking prior to hospitalization and also take the digoxin that was prescribed at the time of discharge.

If the patient does not know they are the same medication, it would not occur to the patient to question the order. In any case, it is not the patient's responsibility to detect this kind of medication error. Proper medication reconciliation by providers before discharge would have prevented such duplication from occurring in the first place.

Throughout a Cycle in Which a Patient Makes Multiple Transitions Between Home and Health Care Organizations

Older adults often go through several transitions during a single episode of care. During each transition, there is potential for breakdown in communications, particularly for patients with multiple comorbidities.[33]

The following factors can contribute to gaps in care during multiple care transitions[34]:
- Poor communication
- Incomplete transfer of information
- Inadequate patient and family education and literacy
- Limited access to necessary services
- Lack of a single "point person" (coordinator) to ensure continuity of care and to become the leader of the team

Practitioners in different settings often act independently of one another. Thus, if they have no knowledge of problems addressed, services provided, test results obtained, or medications prescribed in previous settings, there is potential for overlap or adverse results. Another challenge related to multiple transitions is the tendency of physicians to restrict their practices to a single setting (for example, the office) rather than to follow patients from one setting to the next.[35]

During multiple transitions of care, there is great potential for medical error, service duplication, and inappropriate care, particularly for older patients with multiple comorbidities. Poor transitions can lead to poor patient outcomes, a decrease in patient satisfaction, and an improper use of resources.[35]

References

1. Van Walraven C., et al.: Information exchange among physicians caring for the same patient in the community. *CMAJ* 179:1013–1018, Nov. 2008.

2. Greene B., et al.: How often are physicians and chiropractors provided with patient information when accepting referrals? *J Ambul Care Manage* 30:344–346, Oct.–Dec. 2007.

3. Garåsen H., Johnsen R.: The quality of communication about older patients between hospital physicians and general practitioners: A panel study assessment. *BMC Health Serv Res* 7:133, Aug. 2007.

4. Afilalo M., et al.: Impact of a standardized communication system on continuity of care between family physicians and the emergency department. *CJEM* 9:79–86, Mar. 2007.

5. Lane N., Bragg M.: From emergency department to general practitioner: Evaluating emergency department communication and service to general practitioners. *Emerg Med Australas* 19:346–352, Aug. 2007.

6. Kitch B., et al.: Handoffs causing patient harm: A survey of medical and surgical house staff. *Jt Comm J Qual Patient Saf* 34:563–570, Oct. 2008.

7. Kripalani S., et al.: Deficits in communication and information transfer between hospital-based and primary care physicians: Implications for patient safety and continuity of care. *JAMA* 297:831–841, Feb. 2007.

8. Solet D., et al.: Lost in translation: Challenges and opportunities in physician-to-physician communication during patient handoffs. *Acad Med* 80:1094–1099, Dec. 2005.

9. Poor clinical handover threatening patient care. *Medical News Today,* Mar. 2006. http://www.medicalnewstoday.com/articles/39259.php (accessed Jul. 19, 2010).

10. More shifts mean greater risks in patient handovers, warns MDDUS, Scotland. *Medical News Today,* Apr. 2010. http://www.medicalnewstoday.com/articles/185371.php (accessed Jul. 19, 2010).

11. Amato-Vealey E., Barba M., Vealey R.: Hand-off communication: A requisite for perioperative patient safety. *AORN J* 88:763–770, Nov. 2008.

12. Staggers N., Jennings B.: The content and context of change of shift report on medical and surgical units. *J Nurs Adm* 39:393–398, Sep. 2009.

13. O'Connell B., Penney W.: Challenging the handover ritual: Recommendations for research and practice. *Collegian* 8:14–18, Jul. 2001.

14. Johnson C.: Bad blood: Doctor-nurse behavior problems impact patient care. *Physician Exec* 35:6–11, Nov.–Dec. 2009.

15. Grenny J.: Crucial conversations: The most potent force for eliminating disruptive behavior. *Physician Exec* 35:30–33, Nov.–Dec. 2009.

16. Pronovost P., Vohr E.: *Safe Patients, Smart Hospitals: How One Doctor's Checklist Can Help Us Change Health Care from the Inside Out.* New York City: Hudson Street Press, 2010.

17. Beyea S.: Improving verbal communication in clinical care. *AORN J* 79:1053–1054, 1057, May 2004.

18. Griffin F.: No more "hinting and hoping": Introducing SBAR. *Safer Healthcare.* http://www.saferhealthcare.org.uk/IHI/Topics/ManagingChanging/SafetyStories/SBAR.htm (accessed Oct. 2006).

19. Horowitz L., et al.: Evaluation of an asynchronous physician voicemail sign-out for emergency department admissions. *Ann Emerg Med* 54:368–378, Sep. 2009.

20. Horowitz L., et al.: Dropping the baton: A qualitative analysis of failures during the transition from emergency department to inpatient care. *Ann Emerg Med* 53:701–710, Jun. 2009.

21. Patterson E., Wears R.: Beyond "communication failure." *Ann Emerg Med* 53:711–712, Jun. 2009.

22. Murphy A., Wears R.: The medium is the message: Communication and power in sign-outs. *Ann Emerg Med* 54:379–380, Sep. 2009.

23. McFetridge B., et al.: An exploration of the handover process of critically ill patients between nursing staff from the emergency department and the intensive care unit. *Nurs Crit Care* 12:261–269, Nov.–Dec. 2007.

24. Terrell K., Miller D.: Critical review of transitional care between nursing homes and emergency departments. *Ann Longterm Care* 15, Feb. 1, 2007. http://www.annalsoflongtermcare.com/article/6782 (accessed Jul. 19, 2010).

25. Agency for Healthcare Research and Quality: *HCUP Facts and Figures 2006: Statistics on Hospital-Based Care in the United States.* http://www.hcupus.ahrq.gov/reports/factsandfigures/HAR_2006.pdf (accessed Feb. 25, 2010).

26. Communication with home care staff part of transition. *Healthcare Benchmarks Qual Improv* 16, Mar. 2009. http://findarticles.com/p/articles/mi_m0NUZ/is_2009_March_1/ai_n35568980/ (accessed Feb. 25, 2010).

27. Gandara E., et al.: Communication and information deficits in patients discharged to rehabilitation facilities: An evaluation of five acute care hospitals. *J Hosp Med* 4:E28–E33, Oct. 2009.

28. Rose L., Gerson L., Carbo C.: Transitional care for seriously mentally ill persons: A pilot study. *Arch Psychiatr Nurs* 21:297–308, Dec. 2007.

28. Rands G., et al.: How consultation liaison meetings improved staff knowledge, communication and care. *Nurs Times* 105:18–20, Oct.–Nov. 2009.

30. Tjia J., et al.: Nurse-physician communication in the long-term care setting: Perceived barriers and impact on patient safety. *J Patient Saf* 5:145–152, Sep. 2009.

31. Brown E., et al.: Transition to home care: Quality of mental health, pharmacy, and medical history information. *Int J Psychiatry Med* 36(3):339–349, 2006.

32. Hohl D.: Transitions in home care. *Home Healthc Nurse* 27:499–502, Sep. 2009.

33. Wolff J., et al.: Medicare home health patients' transitions through acute and post-acute care settings. *Med Care* 46:1188–1193, Nov. 2008.

34. Naylor M., Keating S.: Transitional care. *Am J Nurs* 108:58–63, Sep. 2008.

35. American Geriatrics Society: Improving the quality of transitional care for persons with complex care needs. *Assisted Living Consult* pp. 30–32, Mar.–Apr. 2007.

Chapter 2

Patient Experience, Participation, and Understanding of Condition

It is widely understood among health care professionals that patients who are actively involved in their care often enjoy better clinical outcomes.[1] Thus, effective communication between health care providers and patients and their families about all aspects of the patients' care is an important aspect of patient safety. When patients understand what to expect, they are more aware that the choices they make can affect their care, and they are more likely to catch potential errors.[2]

Navigating the health care system can be difficult even under the best of circumstances. When patients are ill, it becomes much more difficult for them to understand their condition and to participate in their care. (*See* Sidebar 2-1 for potential barriers to communication between caregivers and patients.)

Inadequate Patient and Family Preparation at Discharge

Hospital discharge can be a time of increased vulnerability for patients.[3] When patients are discharged, they may not necessarily be in good health. More likely, they are still ill but no longer need such a high level of care.[4] Inadequate patient and family preparation at discharge can lead to a lack of patient understanding of self-care requirements. It can also lead to medication errors, infection, and possible readmission.[5]

The risk of adverse drug events following discharge can be particularly high for elderly patients or those with multiple comorbidities. Lack of effective communication during patient discharge can lead to medication dosing errors, nonadherence, drug interactions, and inadequate monitoring, which in turn can lead to adverse events.[6]

In the fast-paced world of health care, nurses often are working on units that are understaffed and are under pressure to discharge patients "quicker and sicker," so nurses may not have the time they would like to develop detailed discharge plans.[7] However, as technology in hospital care has become

Sidebar 2-1. Potential Barriers to Communication Between Caregivers and Patients

- Resistance of caregivers to change behaviors
- Time pressures from patient care needs and other responsibilities
- Training and time cost of implementing new processes for transitions of care
- Cultural and language differences among patient population and workforce
- Low health literacy
- Lack of financial resources and staffing shortages
- Lack of knowledge about how to improve systems
- Failure of leadership to require implementation of new systems and behaviors
- Lack of information technology infrastructure and interoperability
- Insufficient generally accepted research, data, and economic rationale regarding cost-benefit analysis or return on investment for implementing given recommendations

increasingly sophisticated and length of stay has been greatly reduced, it is more important than ever for patients and families to be adequately prepared for discharge.[8]

A crucial factor in transitions of care at discharge is understanding the environment to which the patient will be returning. It is important to know if that environment can sustain the treatment that has been initiated or if a different environment is required. It is imperative to understand the ability and willingness of the patient's caregiver to provide needed care. It is helpful to understand what services (for example, home care) the patient had prior to admission to the hospital. Care providers from such services can provide critical information that may ease the transition of care. Yet when providers from such services as home care or long term care do try to provide information to the hospital, it sometimes is difficult to find someone who will take the information. And even if someone takes the information, it often either does not get to the right person(s) who can act on it or is not utilized.

Another participation issue involves preparing the patient physically for discharge from the hospital. Such preparation may include some physical therapy to maximize the patient's function and strength prior to leaving the hospital. If the patient seems too weak or frail, caregivers in the receiving environment—particularly family caregivers—may feel overwhelmed or fearful of the patient's incapacity and may simply take the patient back to the hospital rather than attempt to administer care. In some cases, the patient may self-sabotage the transition process because the hospital environment feels "safer" than the environment into which the patient is being transferred. Thus, it is essential that the referral source work with the patient to establish the transition as a desired, mutual goal.

From a practical standpoint, a patient may refuse care by the referral source until insurance authorization is received. Therefore, it is important to allow as much lead time as possible to plan the transition so that there will be no administrative delay in the process.

Preparing the patient and family for discharge is critical to the patient's recovery process. Many practitioners assume that patients understand their discharge instructions. That is a mistake.[3] Sometimes when patients do not understand their discharge instructions, the problem rests with the practitioner. For example, the use of complex medical terms can contribute to a patient's misunderstanding. Written discharge instructions are also often too complex for many patients to comprehend. The average patient reads at an eighth-grade level, yet most discharge instructions are written at a higher level.[3]

In addition to the use of confusing language and difficult-to-comprehend discharge instructions, many other factors affect patients' ability to understand or follow their discharge instructions (*see* Sidebars 2-2 and 2-3).

In some cases, being a member of an ethnic minority group can have an effect on implementation of discharge instructions. For example, in Israel there are differences in the services provided and in implementation of discharge plans between certain

---

Sidebar 2-2. Factors That Affect a Patient's Ability to Understand Discharge Instructions

Reasons that a patient may not understand his or her instructions for discharge include the following:

- Being given much information in a short time
- Illness
- Lack of sleep
- Medication side effects
- Low health literacy
- Limited language proficiency
- Undiagnosed cognitive impairment
- No standardized approach to discharge planning

Source: Adapted from Chugh A., et al.: Better transitions: Improving comprehension of discharge instructions. *Front Health Serv Manage* 25:11–32, Spring 2009.

Sidebar 2-3. Factors That Affect a Patient's Ability to Follow Discharge Instructions

Factors that can affect a patient's ability to follow discharge instructions include the following:

- Lack of social support
- Weekend or holiday discharge (when ancillary support is unavailable)
- Poor medication reconciliation processes
- Depression
- Cognitive impairment
- Functional impairment
- Income

Source: Cumbler E., Carter J., Kutner J.: Failure at the transition of care: Challenges in the discharge of the vulnerable elderly patient. *J Hosp Med* 3:349–352, Jul. 2008.

---

segments of the population (*see* Table 2-1, page 15). One Israeli study showed that Arab patients were less likely than Israeli patients to be referred for long term care or institutional placement, and even when they were referred, they were less likely to actually receive placement.[4] These findings are comparable to those of other minority-group studies.[4]

In the United States, numerous reports have outlined racial and ethnic disparities in all aspects of health care, with

Table 1-1. Factors Related to Implementation of Discharge Plan in Community or Home Care Services

Variable	N	Received Planned Placement N (%)	Odds Ratio	95% GL	p
Total	672	391 (58)			
Age (M = SD)	70.9 = 14.1	73.1 ± 12.4	1.03	1.01–1.04	0.0002
Gender					
Male	264	131 (50)	0.62	0.43–0.50	0.01
Female	408	258 (63)			
Population group					
Arab	79	46 (57)	0.99	0.56–1.74	NS
New immigrant FSU	125	95 (76)	2.67	1.61–4.40	0.01
New immigrant other country	19	11 (58)	1.99	0.72–5.49	NS
Israeli born and veteran resident	449	240 (54)			
Hospital department					
Internal medicine	401	218 (54)	0.55	0.38–0.80	0.002
Surgery	271	173 (64)			
ADL at discharge					
Very limited	236	139 (59)	1.76	1.02–3.04	NS
Needs assistance	350	218 (62)	1.55	0.85–2.81	0.04
Independent	86	34 (40)			
Marital status					
Not married	328	203 (62)	1.02	0.71–1.47	NS
Married	244	188 (55)			
Source of income					
Pension	161	94 (58)	1.61	0.87–2.97	NS
Social security	422	265 (63)	1.73	0.88–3.38	NS
Employment	89	32 (36)			

Source: Auslander G., et al.: Discharge planning in acute care hospitals in Israel: Services planned and levels of implementation and adequacy. *Health Soc Work* 33:178–188, Aug. 2008. Used with permission.

immigrants suffering more adverse patient safety events than patients who were born in the United States.[9,10]

In a study conducted in the Netherlands, the following three key patterns were identified when analyzing patient safety incidents involving immigrants[10]:

1. Inappropriate provider practices related to limited Dutch language proficiency, lack of health insurance, or genetic conditions
2. Differences in perceptions about the patient's illness and treatment expectations
3. Inappropriate treatment due to provider prejudice or stereotyping

Finally, it is important at discharge for providers to confirm where the patient will be, including a valid telephone number at which the patient may be reached. It is extremely frustrating for an agency to which a patient was referred to discover that the patient "cannot be located"—for example, the agency makes repeated calls to the number given but gets no answer or a message that the number has been disconnected, or an agency representative visits the address given but finds no one there. Of course, the person who incurs the greatest loss in this situation is the patient, who is not receiving the recommended care.

Low Health Literacy

Health literacy is the ability to read, understand, and effectively use basic health care instructions and information. Due to the complexity of medical technology and the health system in general, low health literacy can affect anyone of any age, ethnicity, background, or education level.[11] A person may be literate in general but still have low health literacy.

There are two levels of health literacy[12]:
1. *Functional literacy:* the ability to read and comprehend both oral and written materials and to follow caregiver instructions
2. *Conceptual literacy:* the ability not only to read and comprehend instructions but also to be able to evaluate and use that information to make informed decisions

According to the Partnership for Clear Health Communication, the following are characteristics of people with low health literacy[11]:
• Are often less likely to comply with prescribed treatment and self-care regimens.
• Fail to seek preventive care and are at higher (more than double) risk for hospitalization.
• Remain in the hospital nearly two days longer than adults with higher health literacy.
• Often require additional care that results in annual health care costs that are four times higher than for those with higher health literacy skills.

Low health literacy can lead to poor health outcomes, increasing rates of chronic disease, and higher health care costs.[12]

Statistics from the United Nations Educational, Scientific and Cultural Organization Institute of Statistics show that approximately 776 million adults (about 16% of the world's adult population) lack basic literacy skills.[12] More than 89 million people in the United States have limited health literacy.[13] One health literacy survey conducted in the United Kingdom found that among 2,000 survey participants, 1 in 5 had limited health literacy skills.[12] A Canadian study showed that 60% of Canadian adults have limited health literacy skills, and studies from Europe, Australia, and Latin America have reported similar findings.[12]

Health literacy issues and ineffective communication place patients at greater risk of preventable adverse events. If a patient does not understand the implications of his or her diagnosis and the importance of prevention and treatment plans or cannot access health care services because of communication problems, an adverse event may occur. Language and communication barriers—separately or together—have great potential to lead to mutual misunderstandings between patients and their health care providers.

A common cause of a patient's misunderstanding may be a failure to communicate on both sides. On the one hand, physicians often fail to realize that not all patients:
• Understand medical jargon
• Have reading skills that allow them to read or understand forms on their own
• Understand the oral explanations their physicians provide
• Really understand what they have agreed to when they sign consent forms

On the other hand, patients may fail to tell physicians that they do not understand what they have read or heard, may not ask for help interpreting the required forms, and may not always ask questions that would help physicians realize that further explanation is needed. If the cause of a patient's misunderstanding is the failure to communicate clearly and completely on both sides, then the solution must involve both sides. Because physicians have more authority to control communication within the patient-provider relationship, it is up to physicians not only to communicate more clearly and simply with all patients but also to recognize that some patients need more, or different, types of communication to aid their understanding (*see* Chapter 4 for tips for improving effective communication). Health care providers must literally understand where their patients "are coming from"— that is, they must understand the beliefs, values, and cultural mores and traditions that influence how health care information is shared and received.

For people with generally low literacy skills, navigating the health system can be a nightmare. Deciphering hospital signage—such as CARDIAC CATHETERIZATION LABORATORY AND OUTPATIENT RADIOLOGY THIS WAY—completing complex forms, interacting with physicians, following medication instructions, and coping with real or perceived mistreatment by hospital personnel place high demands on those with low literacy skills.[14]

Health care organization leaders are responsible for creating and maintaining cultures of quality and safety. Communication is one of the key systems for which leaders must provide stewardship. Yet, awareness of the prevalence of health literacy issues remains low among health care executives and other managers.

Health care organizations should know and reflect the communities they serve. This knowledge includes not only the primary ethnic groups and languages through which a community expresses itself but also the general literacy level of the community.

Low health literacy can affect informed consent. Consider the two following hypothetical patients. Sixty-one-year-old Hector enters an outpatient clinic for laser surgery to remove cataracts; he has a master's degree in finance and will soon retire from the executive board of a multinational corporation. Forty-three-year-old Michael checks into a community hospital for arthroscopic surgery on his knee; he dropped out of high school but currently manages an auto supply store. Which of these patients would you recommend for a health literacy assessment and targeted education before asking for informed consent? Theoretically, the answer should be both. In reality, it might be neither.[15]

The goal of the informed consent process is to ensure that patients fully understand what actions are being taken to care for them. Rather than simply having a patient sign a piece of paper, the process is meant to consist of a one-on-one discussion between the patient and the physician or other licensed independent practitioner regarding the patient's condition, treatment options (including therapeutic or diagnostic procedures), and possible risks and benefits associated with each option. Only after this discussion has taken place and the patient has been able to ask questions and indicate comprehension of the answers should the consent form be signed.[16]

Even patients who appear to understand the information being communicated may not truly understand. One study found that after agreeing to or receiving care, 18% to 45% of patients were unable to recall the major risks of surgery, 44% did not know the exact nature of their operations, and at least 60% did not read or understand the information contained in informed consent forms even though they signed them.[17] It is estimated that half of all patients do not understand what their physicians have told them. Such patients are not truly informed about the choices they have made.

Making sure that patients understand the information necessary to provide informed consent is a growing challenge. Patients, and often their family members, who do not really grasp what is involved in a care process or procedure may not make the best treatment decisions or may unintentionally do something that contradicts treatment instructions. For example, patients who undergo diagnostic testing using fluoroscopy should understand how long they need to fast before the procedure, which prescribed and over-the-counter (nonprescription) medications may safely be taken, and when those medications may be taken in relation to the procedure. A lack of follow-through on such instructions can delay or prevent the procedure, require a repeat procedure, or, worse, lead to complications during the procedure or misinterpretation of the procedure's results.[15]

Informed consent means helping patients learn everything necessary about their condition or illness and any recommended interventions. "This is as much about communication as it is about consent," says Chandrika Divi, M.P.H., associate project director for The Joint Commission's Center for Patient Safety Research. "That means addressing the patient's educational needs, whether it's taking more time to explain the process or presenting material in a different way."

It is a common belief among health care providers that the use of information technology can improve the overall quality of health care; however, not everyone has access to technology or the ability to comprehend health information once it has been accessed.[18] Many underserved populations—such as ethnic minorities, patients with low socioeconomic status, and those who are not highly educated—do not have computer access or have only limited access.[18] In cases where those populations are able to access health information via computer technology, many have difficulty comprehending the information once it has been accessed because the information is often written at higher reading levels than theirs.[18]

Language Barriers

When the primary language of the patient differs from the primary language of the health care provider and no appropriate interpreter is available, there is great potential for miscommunication. In the United States, more than 55 million people speak a language other than English.[19] In Australia, it is estimated that people speak as many as 100 different languages.[19] In the United Kingdom, more than 300 languages, excluding dialects, have been identified.[19]

About 21 million people in the United States speak English "less than very well."[14] That number is expected to rise in the future. People with limited English proficiency may or may not be highly literate in their own languages. In a growing number of communities, language barriers are a high-priority concern in health care delivery.

A research study conducted by The Joint Commission sought to determine exactly what happens to patients with limited English proficiency in U.S. hospitals. The study examined the characteristics—impact, type, and causes—of adverse events experienced by patients with limited English proficiency and by patients who could communicate well in English.[14]

Among the important findings of the study were the differences in the impact that adverse events had on the two types of patients. Some degree of physical harm occurred to 49.2% of the patients with limited English proficiency who had reported adverse events, but only 29.5% of the patients who spoke English well suffered physical harm from adverse events. Further, among those who did suffer harm, 47% of the patients with limited English proficiency had moderate temporary harm or worse, compared with only 25% of the patients who could speak English well. The rate at which the patients with limited English proficiency suffered permanent or severe harm or death was 3.7%, compared with 1.4% of the patients who spoke English well.[14]

The study does not explain the root cause for these differences. It may be that although all patients are vulnerable to preventable adverse occurrences, patients who are better able to communicate well in English have greater opportunity to participate in their care, to communicate expectations and respond to new information, and to understand when transgressions or variations occur. In other words, they are better prepared to protect themselves.[14]

The goal must be to prevent errors and harm that could occur because of language issues. Since the 1980s, health care organizations and providers have been increasingly relying on interpreters in care encounters. Yet, often the only interpreters available are family members or others who work in the care setting and have some degree of familiarity with the language at hand. This lack of a professional interpreter can place both the patient and the physician or other caregivers in a perilous position, and it is unacceptable. Alice Chen, a physician, wrote of the challenges and frustration she experienced when she had to rely on her patient's husband as the interpreter. Dr. Chen was concerned that her patient's aches, pains, and apparent depression could be the result of spousal abuse, but she was unable to ask about such a possibility with the husband serving as interpreter. Instead, she had to work her way through other possibilities for her patient's condition, without asking what would have been among her first questions.[20]

Limited English proficiency can affect informed consent. The Joint Commission in 2007 reported inconsistent practices in the provision of culturally and linguistically appropriate care. Based on a study of 60 hospitals from across the country, the Joint Commission report stated that although many clinical staff members who were interviewed indicated that they "always use an interpreter for informed consent," others said that their consent form was translated into Spanish but there was no use of an interpreter to discuss the patient's condition and proposed treatment. The use of techniques to verify comprehension, such as "teach back," were used far less often than reliance on a translated form. The Joint Commission report concluded that a "comprehensive approach to meeting the cultural and linguistic, literacy, and other confounding needs of patients is essential to the creation of a health care system that supports informed consent throughout the care process."[21]

References

1. Joint Commission Resources: Patient inclusive care: Encouraging patients to be active participants in their care. *Perspectives on Patient Safety* 5:1–2, 8, Nov. 2005.

2. Joint Commission Resources: Educating patients about infection control: Complying with NPSG.13.01.01.01. *The Joint Commission Perspectives on Patient Safety* 8:10–11, Sep. 2008.

3. Chugh A., et al.: Better transitions: Improving comprehension of discharge instructions. *Front Health Serv Manage* 25:11–32, Spring 2009.

4. Auslander G., et al.: Discharge planning in acute care hospitals in Israel: Services planned and levels of implementation and adequacy. *Health Soc Work* 33:178–188, Aug. 2008.

5. Graham C., Ivey S., Neuhauser L.: From hospital to home: Assessing the transitional care needs of vulnerable seniors. *Gerontologist* 49:23–33, Feb. 2009.

6. Gandara E., et al.: Deficits in discharge documentation in patients transferred to rehabilitation facilities on anticoagulation: Results of a systemwide evaluation. *Jt Comm J Qual Patient Saf* 34:460–463, Aug. 2008.

7. Drury L.: Transition from hospital to home care: What gets lost between the discharge plan and the real world. *J Contin Educ Nurs* 39:198–199, May 2008.

8. Carroll A., Dowling M.: Discharge planning: Communication, education and patient participation. *Brit J Nurs* 16:882–886, Jul.–Aug. 2007.

9. Connecticut Department of Mental Health and Addiction Services: *An Evaluation of Racial and Ethnic Health Disparities in State Inpatient Services.* Jan. 2008. http://www.ct.gov/dmhas/lib/dmhas/oma/disparitiesreport.pdf (accessed Jul. 19, 2010).

10. Suurmond J., et al.: Explaining ethnic disparities in patient safety: A qualitative analysis. *Am J Public Health* 100:S113–S117, Apr. 2010.

11. Partnership for Health Communication at the National Patient Safety Foundation: *Ask Me 3.* http://www.npsf.org/askme3/ (accessed Jul. 19, 2010).

12. Kanj M., Mitic W.: *Promoting Health and Development: Closing the Implementation Gap.* Nairobi, Kenya: 7th Global Conference on Health Promotion, 2009.

13. Kutner M., et al.: *The Health Literacy of America's Adults: Results from the 2003 National Assessment of Adult Literacy.* U.S. Department of Education. Washington, DC: National Center for Education Statistics, Sep. 2006.

14. The Joint Commission: *"What Did the Doctor Say?": Improving Health Literacy to Protect Patient Safety.* 2007. http://www.jointcommission.org/NR/rdonlyres/D5248B2E-E7E6-4121-8874-99C7B4888301/0/improving_health_literacy.pdf (accessed Jul. 19, 2010).

15. Joint Commission Resources: How well informed is your patient's consent? *Perspectives on Patient Safety* 5:1–2, 8, Mar. 2005.

16. Joint Commission Resources: Cultural and linguistic issues in the informed consent process. *The Source* 5:3–4, Jul. 2007.

17. Wilson J.: The crucial link between literacy and health. *Ann Intern Med* 139:875–878, Nov. 2003.

18. Hernandez L.: *Health Literacy, eHealth, and Communication: Putting the Consumer First.* Washington, DC: National Academies Press, 2009.

19. Gil P., et al.: Access to interpreting services in England: Secondary analysis of national data. *BMC Public Health* 9, Jan. 2009. http://www.biomedcentral.com/1471-2458/9/12 (accessed Jul. 19, 2010).

20. Chen A.: Doctoring across the language divide. *Health Aff (Millwood)* 25:803–813, May–Jun. 2006.

21. Wilson-Stronks A., Galvez E.: *Hospitals, Language, and Culture: A Snapshot of the Nation.* Oak Brook, IL: The Joint Commission, 2007.

Chapter 3

Medication Errors

Medications are a primary treatment tool for health care, and the potential for harm to occur from the misuse of medications can carry a significant cost to patients and to society. According to the Sentinel Event Database maintained by The Joint Commission, medication errors are one of the most common causes of sentinel events—unexpected occurrences involving death or serious injury or the risk thereof—reported to The Joint Commission. The database recorded 554 medication errors resulting in death or major injury from 1995 through June 30, 2010.[1]

Medication use is a complex process that is affected by multiple care settings that may or may not be connected, with input from different prescribers. During transitions of care, communication between providers and from provider to patient is often less than ideal, which can lead to an adverse drug event—an injury resulting from a medical intervention related to a medication, including harm from an adverse drug reaction or a medication error.

Medication errors can be categorized as errors of omission or commission. An *error of omission* occurs as a result of an action not taken (for example, when a nurse omits a dose of a medication that should be administered). Or an omission error may involve a patient's condition that remains untreated, such as a diabetic patient with high blood pressure who is not taking an ACE (angiotensin converting enzyme) inhibitor. Errors of omission may or may not lead to adverse outcomes. An *error of commission* occurs as a result of an action taken (for example, when a drug is administered at the wrong time, in the wrong dosage, or using the wrong route) or when a medication is administered that has not been ordered. Both types of errors hold great potential for patient harm.

Many patients have difficulty managing their medications, particularly during transitions of care. Poor communication during transitions of care can lead to problems with medication adherence, potentially resulting in an adverse drug event, readmission to the hospital, or even death. What is needed in these situations but is often missing or lacking is *medication reconciliation*—a formal, standardized process for compiling, recording, and communicating medication information among care providers and the patient.

This chapter includes a discussion of medication-related issues in transitions of care, particularly regarding medication reconciliation, medication administration, and medication adherence.

Medication Reconciliation Issues

Consider the following example from the literature. An 83-year-old man with a history of heart failure arrived at the emergency department with shortness of breath, pain, fever, and lethargy. Due to his altered mental status, the emergency department staff members asked his wife about his medications. She told them that he regularly took several heart medications and a water pill, but she could not recall the specific names or dosages. The patient was diagnosed with and treated for pneumonia. Upon discharge, he was given several new prescriptions. The prescriber did not realize that the patient already had been taking five other prescription medications at home, so the patient was not told to discontinue his home medications. As a result, the patient ended up taking two different doses of furosemide, plus bumetanide, two ACE inhibitors, and two beta blockers after discharge.[2] Clearly, such duplication poses a problem.

The fact that medications need to be reconciled may seem obvious to most organizations, but seemingly simple communications often go awry. Accurate information about patient medication regimens rarely is communicated effectively to and from facilities and local care providers that are not affiliated with those facilities, including the patient's pharmacist.

In September 2004, the U.S. Pharmacopeia added three causes of error to the MEDMARX® reporting program to capture error events involving medication reconciliation failures, allowing for previously unavailable data to be collected about specific causes of medication errors. From September 2004 through July 2008, 11,158 medication errors involving a reconciliation issue were reported to MEDMARX.[3] Of those, 52% of reconciliation errors occurred during admission, 39% during the patient's transition or transfer to another level of care, and 9% at discharge. More than 40% of the "admission" and "transition" errors were intercepted before reaching the patient, but only 25% of discharge reconciliation errors were intercepted. Ineffective communication was once again identified as a major problem area.

Awareness of the importance of medication reconciliation is growing worldwide as increasing numbers of individual health care facilities adopt a medication reconciliation process. Among the nine Patient Safety Solutions approved by the World Health Organization Collaborating Centre for Patient Safety Solutions (which includes The Joint Commission and Joint Commission International) in 2007 was a solution for assuring medication accuracy at transitions in care.[4] This solution focused attention on the risk of nonreconciled medications and the value of a medication reconciliation process.

Medication reconciliation can help prevent such errors as the following:
- Failure to continue needed home medications while in the hospital
- Failure to discontinue home medications that are contraindicated while in the hospital
- Failure to discontinue one medication when an equivalent medication is ordered
- Failure to modify route and dosages when needed
- Erroneous changes in dosing when medications are continued from the home or into the hospital
- Missed or duplicated doses resulting from inaccurate medication records
- Failure to discontinue certain medications at discharge
- Failure to specify which home medications should be resumed at home after discharge
- Transcription errors that result from having to rewrite orders at every transfer point

In an age of specialization, often no one physician is reviewing the medication list, including the patient's over-the-counter medications, in its totality. This situation may be partially due to the patient's not communicating all these medications properly. Even in organizations that do a good job of reconciling orders upon admission and discharge, some providers do not adequately educate patients about their medications. Patients often do not have a clear understanding of which medications they are being given when hospitalized or how their medication regimens change on a day-to-day basis. They are then left to figure it out when they get home. Medication reconciliation greatly improves provider transmission of information. Keeping patients engaged and educated throughout the process helps ensure their safety and maximize their understanding of their medication regimens.

Medication Administration Issues

When you consider that between 50 and 100 steps are involved in the process of providing a new medication to a patient from the time the order is written to the time that the medication is administered to the patient, it is not surprising that medication errors are relatively common.[5] Recent statistics show that 38% of medication errors occur during medication administration. Although 39% of medication errors occur during prescribing and 14% during dispensing, pharmacists and nurses intercept about 40% of prescribing errors and nurses intercept about 40% of dispensing errors before they reach the patient.[5] However, only 2% of administration errors are intercepted before reaching the patient because they occur at the end of the process.[5]

The most common cause of medication administration error is performance deficit, which is defined as "a cause that results when the person involved had the requisite knowledge and training to perform the necessary task but failed to do so."[6] Other causes of medication administration error include not following procedure or protocol, knowledge deficit, inadequate monitoring, poor communication, and improper use of intravenous infusion pumps.[6]

Other factors that may contribute to medication administration errors include the following[5-7]:
- Work-load increase
- Insufficient training
- Lack of standardized medication administration processes
- Stress
- Fatigue
- Interruptions or distractions

Studies have clearly demonstrated that frequent interruptions can lead to errors.[8] Nurses are often interrupted, sometimes several times, when preparing and administering medications.[7] Interruptions can come from many different sources, such as patients, visitors, other nurses, ancillary staff, physicians, and other clinical staff. Medication administration also may be interrupted by the need for the nurse to clarify or correct medication orders.[7] During one observation, a nurse was interrupted 11 times while attempting to prepare and administer a medication.[7] Not only do interruptions increase the risk for error, but the more interruptions that occur, the longer the process takes (*see* Figure 3-1, page 24).

Medication Adherence Issues

As described in the literature, an 86-year-old woman with a history of mild dementia, major depression with psychotic features, and multiple comorbidities was admitted to a hospital after her congestive heart failure worsened. After her condition stabilized, she was discharged on a holiday weekend with multiple new prescriptions but no way to pick them up. Her family was out of town for the holiday and could not be reached.[9] How could such a patient be expected to take her medications properly?

Immediately after discharge from a hospital, the risk of an adverse drug event greatly increases. The period after hospital discharge can be a vulnerable time for patients as they resume responsibility for their own care. However, hospital discharges frequently are rushed, which can result in the patient's misunderstanding the treatment plan.[10]

Postdischarge medication adherence issues include the following[10]:
- Failure to fill prescriptions
- Misunderstanding about how to take the medications
- Discrepancies between what the patient is supposed to be taking and what he or she is actually taking

Studies show that elderly patients and patients who are taking six or more medications are more likely than other patients to experience medication-related problems after discharge.[10] Adverse drug events also are more common in patients who are taking high-alert medications such as anticoagulants, insulin, and certain cardiac medications.[10]

In addition to adverse drug events, nonadherence to medication regimens can result in a worsening of the disease for which the patient was originally hospitalized.[11] Mortality rates also are higher in cases of nonadherence.[10] Sidebar 3-1 lists types of medication nonadherence.

Reasons for medication nonadherence include the following[10–12]:
- Medication costs

Sidebar 3-1. Types of Medication Nonadherence

Nonadherence to medication regimens can take many forms, including the following:
- Forgetting to take a medication
- Skipping a dose
- Not taking the medication when feeling better
- Not taking the medication when feeling ill
- Forgetting to take doses of medications that should be taken more than once a day
- Not taking the medication because of side effects
- Not taking the medication because it does not seem to be helping
- Changing the dose to suit own needs

Source: Kripalani S., et al.: Medication use among inner-city patients after hospital discharge: Patient-reported barriers and solutions. *Mayo Clin Proc* 83:529–535, May 2008.

- Lack of outside support
- Ineffective communication between provider and patient

Medication Costs

It is estimated that about 20% of prescriptions given at discharge are never filled.[12] In one study among inner-city patients, only 40% of the respondents had filled their prescriptions the day they were discharged. An additional 20% filled their prescriptions one or two days after discharge, and 18% waited from three to nine days to get their prescriptions filled.[11] When asked why they would delay filling their prescriptions, more than one-third of the respondents admitted that cost was an issue.[11]

Prescriptions given at discharge can be a large unexpected expense, particularly for patients who are on a fixed income.[6] Many patients simply cannot afford their medications; others admit to taking less than the prescribed dose to make the medications last longer.[10,12]

Physicians often do not know the cost of the medications they are prescribing, and many physicians may not think to ask patients whether cost is a factor. Many physicians also may not be aware of formulary restrictions and tiered costs, which are common in the United States, Canada, Australia, New Zealand, Singapore, and some European countries.[12] If that information is not available and used to guide prescribing, the result can be higher out-of-pocket costs

Figure 3-1. Effect of Interruptions on Medication Administration Process Flow

Based on a study conducted at Sharp Grossmont Hospital in La Mesa, California, this flow map illustrates a medication administration process used in a hospital setting. When there are no interruptions, following the path shown by the solid lines and arrows, the process takes an average time of 7 minutes. But when there are interruptions, following the path shown by the broken lines and arrows, the average time nearly triples, increasing to 20 minutes.

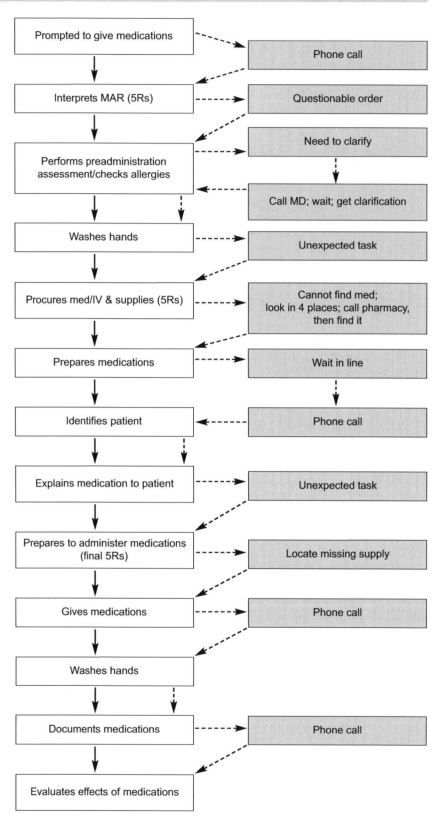

Source: Adapted from Conrad C., et al.: Medication room madness: Calming the chaos. *J Nurs Care Qual* 25(2):137–144, 2010.

for patients,[12] which in turn can increase the likelihood of nonadherence.

Lack of Social or Other Outside Support

Patients often are discharged from the hospital with a variety of new self-care needs that must be met, including a new medication regimen. If the patient has no social or ancillary support, he or she may find it difficult to meet those needs, particularly if the patient has a cognitive or functional impairment.[12]

Transportation also can be a problem for patients with no social or other outside support. Many such patients have difficulty getting to the pharmacy to fill their prescriptions. Some of these patients also may have difficulty finding transportation to their follow-up appointments. As a result, adherence issues for such patients could remain undetected for a long time.

Ineffective Communication Between Provider and Patient

Difficulty managing medications, particularly after hospital discharge, often is related to poor communication. Patients are given much information in a short time just prior to discharge, and some of this information contains complex medical jargon.[12] In one study, 18% of patients with medication adherence issues reported not understanding how to take their new medications. The same study showed that 71% of patients who had issues with medication adherence reported that they did not have a clear understanding of the purpose of their discharge medications.[11] In many instances, physicians may overestimate how much of the information that they have given their patients is actually comprehended; therefore, physicians often do not give patients and family enough time to ask questions.[12] Low health literacy, language barriers, and cultural differences also may contribute to limited comprehension of medication regimens and medication nonadherence.[12]

References

1. The Joint Commission: *Sentinel Event Statistics as of: June 30, 2010.* http://www.jointcommission.org/NR/rdonlyres/377FF7E7-F565-4D61-9FD2-593CA688135B/0/SE_Stats_9_09.pdf (accessed Aug. 25, 2010).

2. Young B.: Medication reconciliation matters. *Medsurg Nurs* 17:332–336, Oct. 2008.

3. Diane D. Cousins, e-mail message to Meghan Pillow, Nov. 4, 2008.

4. WHO Collaborating Centre for Patient Safety Solutions: Assuring medication accuracy at transitions in care. *Patient Safety Solutions* 1(solution 6), May 2007. http://www.ccforpatientsafety.org/common/pdfs/fpdf/presskit/PS-Solution6.pdf (accessed Jul. 19, 2010).

5. Kliger J., et al.: Empowering frontline nurses: A structured intervention enables nurses to improve medication administration accuracy. *Jt Comm J Qual Patient Saf* 35:604–612, Dec. 2009.

6. Santell J., Cousins D.: Medication errors involving wrong administration technique. *Jt Comm J Qual Patient Saf* 31:528–532, Sep. 2005.

7. Conrad C., et al.: Medication room madness: Calming the chaos. *J Nurs Care Qual* 25:137–144, Apr.–Jun. 2010.

8. Westbrook J., et al.: Association of interruptions with an increased risk and severity of medication administration errors. *Arch Intern Med* 170:683–690, Apr. 2010.

9. Cumbler E., Carter J., Kutner J.: Failure at the transition of care: Challenges in the discharge of the vulnerable elderly patient. *J Hosp Med* 3:349–352, Jul. 2008.

10. Kripalani S., et al.: Frequency and predictors of prescription-related issues after hospital discharge. *J Hosp Med* 3:12–19, Jan. 2008.

11. Kripalani S., et al.: Medication use among inner-city patients after hospital discharge: Patient-reported barriers and solutions. *Mayo Clin Proc* 83:529–535, May 2008.

12. Cua Y., Kripalani S.: Medication use in the transition from hospital to home. *Ann Acad Med Singapore* 37:136–141, Feb. 2008.

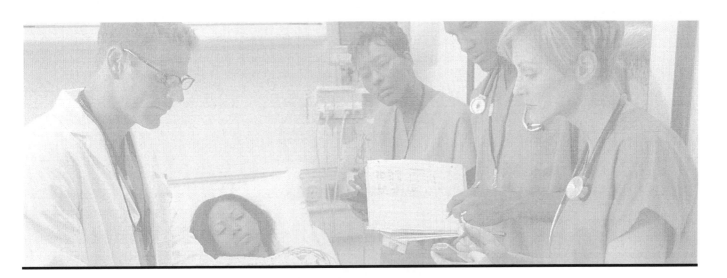

Part 2

Solutions for
Coordinating and Standardizing Communication During Transitions of Care

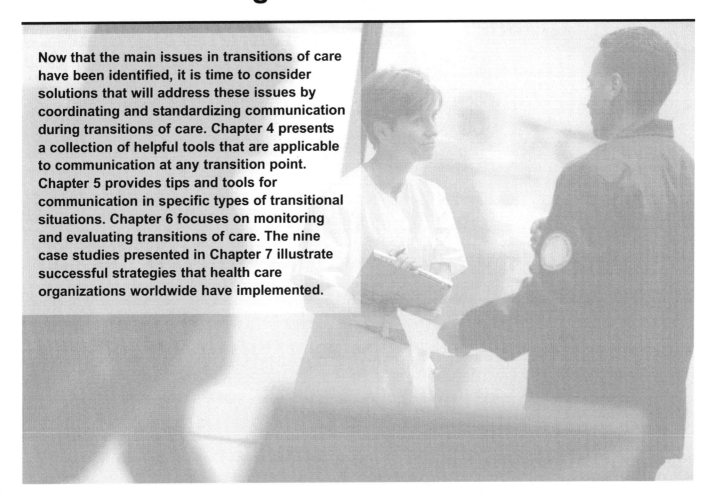

Now that the main issues in transitions of care have been identified, it is time to consider solutions that will address these issues by coordinating and standardizing communication during transitions of care. Chapter 4 presents a collection of helpful tools that are applicable to communication at any transition point. Chapter 5 provides tips and tools for communication in specific types of transitional situations. Chapter 6 focuses on monitoring and evaluating transitions of care. The nine case studies presented in Chapter 7 illustrate successful strategies that health care organizations worldwide have implemented.

Chapter 4

Tools Applicable to Communication at Any Transition Point

To address the issues in transitions of care discussed in Part 1, a number of organizations, including The Joint Commission, have developed communication tools for any transition point. This chapter discusses in detail some of the tools used by The Joint Commission and Joint Commission International (JCI). Available forms, checklists, and other tools are provided as examples.

Tracer Methodology

Tracer methodology can be an effective way to monitor transition-of-care processes. For both The Joint Commission and JCI, tracer methodology is at the foundation of the on-site survey experience. The following information regarding communication requirements for specific accreditation programs was provided by surveyors. Tracer scenarios are also provided for each program type.

Ambulatory Care and Office-Based Surgery

During an ambulatory care survey, Michael Jarema, M.B.A., Joint Commission field representative, Ambulatory Care, expects to see standardized transition-of-care processes throughout the organization. (The Joint Commission uses the title *field representative* for what JCI calls a *surveyor.*) He looks to see whether the organization has given careful consideration to identifying the transitions of care that occur in the care of the patient and that the organization has implemented standardized processes for each transition of care. "For example, if a physician, nurse, or midwife is going on vacation, and during his or her absence will be transferring care to another provider, I would want to know what the organization's process is for consistently communicating information between providers," he says. "Is complete information being consistently communicated among all caregivers to ensure patient safety and continuity of care?"

Jarema says he surveyed one organization that had studied transitions of care as part of its annual proactive risk assessment by using a failure mode and effects analysis

(FMEA). The organization tracked patients through multiple levels of care using a flowchart and then assessed each point where patient information and responsibility for the patient's care were transferred. "They began at registration and continued to follow the patient through the referral process at discharge," he says. This exercise allowed the organization to identify breakdowns in communication and to standardize the communication expectations during each transition of care.

When conducting a survey, Jarema reviews patient charts, paying particular attention to notes between providers. "I want to know what information was exchanged when there was a change or delegation of responsibility for the patient's care," he says. Jarema also talks to physicians and other care providers and asks them how information was exchanged during the transition of care. "What I'm looking for is a consistent process," he says. "Individual pieces of information will change for each specific patient, but a consistent, overarching approach to the sharing and communication of information should be in place."

Behavioral Health Care

Gale Levesque, Ph.D., Joint Commission field representative, Behavioral Health, observes transitions of care during shift change when surveying behavioral health facilities that operate around the clock, such as shelters or group homes. "There's usually a 15-minute overlap during change of shift, so I sit in the room and see what's being communicated," Levesque says. "Twenty-four-hour facilities also have continuous communication logs where they record significant events. I like to review those, too."

Levesque monitors communication at other types of behavioral health facilities by communicating with the client's primary therapist or case worker. "Clients are often being seen by more than one facility, but there is usually one person who receives all of the client's information and integrates it into a summary note," says Levesque. "Once a month, representatives from all facilities get together for a treatment plan review. That's where everything comes together."

The following example, provided by Levesque, is a potential tracer scenario in behavioral health: "You might have a person who lives in a group home but who also goes to a day program. Because a lot of the communication between facilities is verbal, I might go to the day program and ask them how they would communicate with the group home if the client was involved in an altercation at the program. Then I would go to the group home and ask them what type of information they receive from the day program when that type of incident occurs."

Hospital and Critical Access Hospital

When surveying a hospital, Alan Funtanilla, R.N., M.S., Joint Commission field representative, Hospital, looks for standardized transitions of care between all staff members involved in those transitions. According to Funtanilla, many hospitals do not yet have standardized approaches for communication between physicians or for communication between nurses and ancillary personnel.

During a hospital survey, Funtanilla also observes transitions of care to see whether providers are given an opportunity for questions and have the ability to verify information received during a transition of care. "I'm looking to see if they have a standardized approach," he says, "and whether or not they use techniques such as read-backs to verify information."

Deborah Pellini, R.N, M.S., Joint Commission field representative, Hospital, uses a similar approach. "There are several things I want to know when doing a survey," she says. "First of all, do they have a standardized methodology? What is the overall conceptual framework that they're using? If they have developed a specific tool, who is using it?" According to Pellini, some hospitals she has surveyed have standardized approaches only for nurses, and others have processes only for physicians, transporters, or other ancillary staff. "If a standardized approach is being used, I would want to see that it's been customized for use not only for nurses at shift change but for communication between departments as well." Pellini says she would also like to see the standardized methodology used consistently. "I continue to see inconsistencies within nursing staffs during transitions of care," she says.

According to Pellini, another risk point is when transitions occur between an individual who uses a "hard copy" medical record (that is, on paper only) and an individual who has access to an electronic medical record (EMR). "Even when transitions occur between two units that have an EMR, consistency in the utility of the screen within the EMR for transitions of care may vary," she says.

When tracing a patient in a hospital, Funtanilla goes to a unit and asks whether any patients are getting ready to be transferred. For example, he might go to a telemetry unit and ask to trace a patient who is being transferred to the intensive care unit (ICU). He then follows the patient through the transition-of-care process until the patient has been admitted to the accepting unit.

When Pellini traces a hospital patient, she goes to a unit, chooses a patient, and then finds the assigned nurse and inquires about the patient's point of entry. For example, if the patient was transferred to the intensive care unit from the emergency department, Pellini would ask the nurse how the transition of care was conducted. "I would also want to know how information is communicated at shift change, what would be communicated if the patient was transferred from the ICU to a step-down unit, and even what is communicated to a covering nurse during breaks," she says. Pellini also observes transitions of care when feasible.

Home Care

When conducting a home care survey, Suzan Lambert, M.S., R.N., B.C., Joint Commission field representative, Home Care, looks for standardization to see whether the same information is shared regardless of who is involved in the transition of care. "Whoever is taking over the patient needs to have all pertinent information as to what is going on with the patient on that particular day," she says. "There also has to be a method for that person to ask questions about the patient and the plan of care."

Lambert admits that the home care setting makes it challenging to survey transitions of care. "The patient isn't physically there, so you can't do walking rounds," she says. "You have to talk to the staff to see what type of exchange is occurring between the person giving up the patient and the person who is receiving the patient. For example, if a nurse is on call, how does he or she get information about each patient, and how can he or she get additional information, if needed?"

In home care, the patient's care is transferred from the primary nurse to another nurse for the weekend. "If a patient is receiving daily wound care or IV [intravenous] therapy, someone has to pick up care for that patient when the primary nurse is not working," Lambert says. When surveying this type of transition of care, Lambert talks to both the primary nurse and the receiving nurse to find out what type of information is being shared. "I particularly want to make sure that both are aware of the patient's diagnosis, what types of medications the patient is taking, and the patient's response to those medications," she says. "I also want to know where they are in the process of teaching the patient and family what the caregivers need to know to continue care around the clock."

When tracing a home care patient, Lambert also asks the patient or caregiver whether staff members seem prepared when they visit. "Patients and caregivers can generally let me know if staff is aware of the purpose of the visit and what they need to do to get their jobs done," she says. "I ask how easy it is for the patient when someone new comes to provide care. Does this new staff person seem to know why he or she is there and what needs to be done for the patient?"

Laboratory

One of the first questions Kathleen Cross, M.T. (A.S.C.P.), Joint Commission field representative, Laboratory, wants answered during a laboratory survey is: Who is responsible for making sure the physician receives test results in a timely manner? "If a test takes longer than a day, that can sometimes be a problem, particularly if the patient goes home," she says. "However, the use of electronic medical records is making this less of an issue, especially in systems that provide all physicians with access from their offices."

Cross has surveyed more than 300 laboratories and has found that the processes differ, depending on the hospital. "Sometimes the lab is responsible for forwarding results to the physician, sometimes it's left up to the nurse, and sometimes it's up to medical records personnel," she says. "Being a lab person myself, my preference is that the lab take responsibility."

"I recently traced a patient from an outpatient clinic to a children's hospital," says Cross. "There was contact from physician to physician and from nurse to nurse. In addition, emergency medical services called the hospital twice while en route to give them an update. It was very well done."

Long Term Care

Long term care surveyors are often particularly interested in how information is communicated concerning residents with dementia. According to Carol Johnson, Joint Commission field representative, Long Term Care, some long term care facilities have developed communication tools that convey special needs to the facility that is receiving the resident. These tools help caregivers communicate not only with one another but also with the resident. Some of the information provided by these tools may include the following:

- Information about activities of daily living
- How much help the resident needs
- What name the resident responds to
- What types of behaviors the resident is exhibiting
- How those behaviors can best be managed

When tracing a long term care resident, the surveyor might talk to each caregiver and ask what information is being transferred during a transition of care. "This is particularly important if a resident has an infection and is on contact precautions," Johnson says. "I might check with everyone who came in contact with that resident and find out how they learned that the resident was on contact precautions."

The Situation–Background–Assessment–Recommendation (SBAR) Technique

Many health care organizations have adopted the Situation–Background–Assessment–Recommendation (SBAR) technique to help them standardize their processes for transitions of care. The SBAR technique was originally used by the U.S. military for nuclear submarines. A patient safety team from Kaiser Permanente in Oakland, California, developed a health care version of this technique to facilitate communication between physicians and nurses.[1] The Kaiser Permanente SBAR form is shown in Figure 4-1, page 32. Kaiser also has developed Guidelines for Communicating with Physicians Using the SBAR Process (*see* Figure 4-2, page 33).

When using the SBAR technique, the following information is transferred between caregivers during transitions of care:
1. *Situation:* What is going on with the patient?
2. *Background:* What is the clinical background or context?
3. *Assessment:* What do I think the problem is?
4. *Recommendation:* What would I do to correct it?

For step-by-step instructions on how to use the SBAR technique, *see* Sidebar 4-1, page 34.

Figure 4-1. SBAR Report to Physician About a Critical Situation

S	**Situation**
	I am calling about <u>\<patient name and location\></u>.
	The patient's code status is <u>\<code status\></u>
	The problem I am calling about is _____.
	    I am afraid the patient is going to arrest.
	
	I have just assessed the patient personally:
	
	Vital signs are: Blood pressure _____/_____, Pulse _____, Respiration_____ and temperature _____
	
	I am concerned about the:
	    Blood pressure because it is over 200 or less than 100 or 30 mmHg below usual
	    Pulse because it is over 140 or less than 50
	    Respiration because it is less than 5 or over 40.
	    Temperature because it is less than 96 or over 104.

B	**Background**
	The patient's mental status is:
	    Alert and oriented to person place and time.
	    Confused and cooperative or non-cooperative
	    Agitated or combative
	    Lethargic but conversant and able to swallow
	    Stuporous and not talking clearly and possibly not able to swallow
	    Comatose. Eyes closed. Not responding to stimulation.
	The skin is:
	    Warm and dry
	    Pale
	    Mottled
	    Diaphoretic
	    Extremities are cold
	    Extremities are warm
	The patient is not or is on oxygen.
	    The patient has been on _____ (l/min) or (%) oxygen for _____ minutes (hours)
	    The oximeter is reading _____%
	    The oximeter does not detect a good pulse and is giving erratic readings.

A	**Assessment**
	    This is what I think the problem is: <u>\<say what you think is the problem\></u>
	    The problem seems to be cardiac infection neurologic respiratory _____
	    I am not sure what the problem is but the patient is deteriorating.
	    The patient seems to be unstable and may get worse, we need to do something.

R	**Recommendation**
	I suggest or request that you <u>\<say what you would like to see done\></u>.
	    transfer the patient to critical care
	    come to see the patient at this time.
	    Talk to the patient or family about code status.
	    Ask the on-call family practice resident to see the patient now.
	    Ask for a consultant to see the patient now.
	Are any tests needed:
	    Do you need any tests like CXR, ABG, EKG, CBC, or BMP?
	    Others?
	If a change in treatment is ordered then ask:
	    How often do you want vital signs?
	    How long to you expect this problem will last?
	    If the patient does not get better when would you want us to call again?

This figure provides an example of one way the SBAR technique can be used to facilitate communication with a physician.

Source: Kaiser Permanente: *SBAR Report to Physician About a Critical Situation.* Available at www.IHI.org.
This SBAR tool was developed by Kaiser Permanente. Please feel free to use and reproduce these materials in the spirit of patient safety, and please retain this footer in the spirit of appropriate recognition.

Figure 4-2. Guidelines for Communicating with Physicians Using the SBAR Process

1. **Use the following modalities according to physician preference, if known. Wait no longer than five minutes between attempts.**
   1. Direct page (if known)
   2. Physician's call service
   3. During weekdays, the physician's office directly
   4. On weekends and after hours during the week, physician's home phone
   5. Cell phone

   Before assuming that the physician you are attempting to reach is not responding, utilize all modalities.
   For emergent situations, use appropriate resident service as needed to ensure safe patient care.

2. **Prior to calling the physician, follow these steps:**
   - Have I seen and assessed the patient myself before calling?
   - Has the situation been discussed with resource nurse or preceptor?
   - Review the chart for appropriate physician to call.
   - Know the admitting diagnosis and date of admission.
   - Have I read the most recent MD progress notes and notes from the nurse who worked the shift ahead of me?
   - Have available the following when speaking with the physician:
     – Patient's chart
     – List of current medications, allergies, IV fluids, and labs
     – Most recent vital signs
     – Reporting lab results: provide the date and time test was done and results of previous tests for comparison
     – Code status

3. **When calling the physician, follow the SBAR process:**
   (S) Situation: What is the situation you are calling about?
   - Identify self, unit, patient, room number.
   - Briefly state the problem, what is it, when it happened or started, and how severe.

   (B) Background: Pertinent background information related to the situation could include the following:
   - The admitting diagnosis and date of admission
   - List of current medications, allergies, IV fluids, and labs
   - Most recent vital signs
   - Lab results: provide the date and time test was done and results of previous tests for comparison
   - Other clinical information
   - Code status

   (A) Assessment: What is the nurse's assessment of the situation?

   (R) Recommendation: What is the nurse's recommendation or what does he/she want? Examples:
   - Notification that patient has been admitted
   - Patient needs to be seen now
   - Order change

4. **Document the change in the patient's condition and physician notification.**

These guidelines provide a detailed explanation of one way to use the SBAR technique in a health care setting.

Source: Kaiser Permanente: *Guidelines for Communicating with Physicians Using the SBAR Process.* Available at www.IHI.org.
This SBAR tool was developed by Kaiser Permanente. Please feel free to use and reproduce these materials in the spirit of patient safety, and please retain this footer in the spirit of appropriate recognition.

Sidebar 4-1. The SBAR Technique, Step-by-Step

When calling the physician, use the SBAR process as follows:

Situation: What is the situation you are calling about?
• Identify yourself, the unit, the patient, and the room number.
• Briefly state the problem: what it is, when it started, and the severity.

Background: Provide background information relevant to the situation, which may include the following:
• The patient's chart
• The admitting diagnosis and date and time of admission
• A list of current medications, allergies, intravenous fluids, and labs
• The most recent vital signs
• Lab results, with the date and time each test was performed and results of previous tests for comparison
• Other clinical information
• Code status

Assessment: What is your assessment of the situation?

Recommendation: What is your recommendation or what do you want?
Examples include the following:
• Patient to be admitted
• Patient to be seen now
• Order to be changed

Source: Joint Commission Resources: The SBAR technique: Improves communication, enhances patient safety. *Perspectives on Patient Safety* 5:1–2, 8, Feb. 2005.

The SBAR technique was originally designed for communication in high-risk situations between nurses and physicians; however, organizations today are adapting it for use during all types of communication. For example, at Kaiser, the SBAR technique is used not only for communication between caregivers but also in leadership reports, e-mails, and voice-mail messages.

Implementing SBAR

Before adopting the SBAR technique or any other standardized process for transitions of care, organizations need to solicit input from key stakeholders and allow them the opportunity to help design the processes. It is much easier to implement a new process if those who will be using it are involved so they can ensure that the new process is compatible with current work-flow patterns.

Doctors Hospital, an acute care facility in Coral Gables, Florida, that is part of the not-for-profit health care system Baptist Health South Florida, adopted the SBAR technique

as its framework for the development of standardized forms for transitions of care. Using the SBAR technique, the hospital system developed two nursing tools, which were then pilot tested by staff members of units who volunteered to try them. Based on input from the nurses, the hospital's multidisciplinary team of health care professionals was able to determine which tool was more user-friendly (*see* Figure 4-3, page 35). After the initial nursing form was released for use on medical/surgical nursing units, the team began working on developing additional tools that were tailored to other types of transitions of care. For an example of such a tool, *see* Figure 4-4, page 36. For a sample form to use for transitions of care within ambulatory care facilities, *see* Figure 4-5, page 37.

One disadvantage of the SBAR technique is that nurses sometimes initially find it difficult to make recommendations for a patient's care to a physician because they have been taught not to make medical diagnoses; however, nurses should be encouraged to make recommendations because the

Figure 4-3. Handoff Report: Nurse

🍍 Doctors Hospital
BAPTIST
HEALTH

NURSE: _____   DATE: _____

SITUATION BACKGROUND	Consulting MD's:	Labs & Critical Values:	Admission:
LABEL		H/H: _____	Date & Time _____
	Other consults: PT / OT / SWS	BMP: _____	Complete / Pending Admission Assessment Form (Yellow)
Diagnosis:	**Diet:**	PT: _____	SOC Advance Directives
	Tube Feedings: _____	INR: _____	Education Form (Purple) Admission Med Reconciliation Patient Belongings Form
		PTT: _____	
	Fluid Restriction & how much:	MD Called? Yes No	
History & Surgeries:	**Activity:**	**Surgery/Procedure Today:**	
		Consent/Checklist done? Yes No	**RECOMMENDATION/NOTES:**
	Falls Risk: Yes No Hx falling: Yes No Morse Fall Score: _____	**Meds & Treatments Today:**	
	Alarms: Yes No	_____	
	Companion: Yes No	_____	
Allergies:	Advance Directive/DNR: Yes No	_____	
VS q: _____		_____	
		IV fluids:	
Daily wt: _____	Mini Lift:		
Neuro checks q: _____		Blood:	
Foley: _____			
I&O: _____	**Precautions:**	PCA:	
O2: NC / Mask / Treatments:	Decubitis / Aspiration / Seizure	**ASSESSMENTS:**	
Accucheck q: _____	Bleeding / Total Hip / Total Knee	Head / Neuro	
	Isolation: Type _____	Skin	
SCD's: Yes No		Cardiac/Tele	
Drains:		Resp	
Dressings:		GI/GU	
		Ortho	
Discharge Planning:		IV site / tubing	

NOT PART OF MEDICAL RECORD

This report is used by a nurse preparing a patient for a transition of care.

Source: Doctors Hospital, Baptist Health South Florida, Coral Gables, Florida. Used with permission.

Figure 4-4. Nurse Handoff Communication: Intensive Care Unit/Primary Care Unit

Date: _____

Room #	Name/Age: Label Allergies:	Neuro:	GCS:
Situation/Diagnosis:		Cardiac:	
Back Ground/History:		Respiratory:	
Assessment/Lines/ IV:		GI:	
Diagnostics:		GU:	
Recommendation/Pending/ Miscellaneous: Consults: Results: Labs: Paperwork Pending:		Skin:	
		Accuchecks:	Code Status:

NOT PART OF THE MEDICAL RECORD

This report is used by nurses for a patient's transition of care between an intensive care unit and a primary care unit.

Source: Doctors Hospital, Baptist Health South Florida, Coral Gables, Florida. Used with permission.

Figure 4-5. Handoff Communication: Ambulatory Care

Date:_____ **Time:**_____ **Patient's name:** **PACU nurse:** **Surgeon:** **Anesthesia:** **Report given to:**_____	Dressings:_____ _____ Peri pad:_____ Drains:_____ Compresses:_____ Elevation:_____	Labs & procedures today: H/H:_____ BMP:_____ PT:_____ INR:_____ PTT:_____ Other:_____	Medication reconciliation Complete / Pending Critical Values:_____ _____ _____ _____ _____
Situation/Background _____ _____ _____ Allergies:_____ BP_____ Temp:_____ P_____ Resp_____ SAO2_____ RA_____ 02 liters_____	Ortho: Ice:_____ Ace wrap:_____ Sling:_____ Brace:_____ CPM:_____ Hot ice:_____ P.T._____	_____ _____ _____ _____ _____ _____ _____ _____	Notes:_____ _____ _____ _____ _____ _____ _____ _____
Nausea:_____ Meds for nausea:_____ _____ Pain level:_____ Site of pain:_____ Meds given in PACU:_____ _____ RX on chart _____	Precautions: Falls Risk:_____ Seizure precaution _____ CMS:_____ Treatments:_____ Blood sugar: _____ SCDs:_____	Other medications: _____ _____ _____ _____ _____ Treatments:_____ _____ _____ _____	_____ _____ _____ _____ _____ _____ _____ _____
Intake and output: Oral:_____ IV fluids:_____ _____ Bag number:_____ Void/foley_____ Diet:_____	Assessments: Neuro_____ Cardiac:_____ Resp:_____ GI:_____ GU:_____ IV Site:_____	Recommendations: _____ _____ _____ _____ _____ _____	Time transferred to floor:_____ Report to:_____ Report from:_____

This report is used for a patient's transition of care in an ambulatory care facility.

Source: Doctors Hospital, Baptist Health South Florida, Coral Gables, Florida. Used with permission.

nurses are the ones in the position to know what is happening with the patient at the time. The ultimate decision regarding what should be done for the patient remains with the physician.

Many organizations that have implemented the SBAR technique have discovered that, contrary to what they feared, physicians did not react negatively to recommendations from nurses. Some physicians actually welcomed the recommendations and expressed frustration when nurses were not straightforward about what was going on with their patients.[2]

Transition Scenarios Using the SBAR Technique

Table 4-1, page 39, provides examples of how to use the SBAR technique during specific patient scenarios. These scenarios and SBAR examples were developed by Jeff L. Convissar, M.D., practice leader, National Risk Management, Kaiser Permanente, Oakland, California, and Paul Preston, M.D., staff anesthesiologist, San Francisco Kaiser Permanente Medical Center, San Francisco, and regional safety educator, Permanente Medical Group, San Francisco. When training staff members to use the SBAR technique, organizations can create their own patient scenarios and ask staff members to demonstrate how to use the SBAR technique for each scenario.

The Transitional Care Model

The Transitional Care Model, which was developed by the University of Pennsylvania School of Nursing, is a multidisciplinary model of care designed to improve transitions of care for chronically ill or hospitalized patients. It includes both in-hospital care planning and home follow-up care. The model includes 10 key elements[3]:

1. A transitional care nurse, who is the patient's primary care coordinator
2. In-hospital assessment, preparation, and development of an evidence-based plan of care
3. Regular home visits by the transitional care nurse and ongoing 24-hour telephone support
4. Facilitation of continuity of care between the hospital and the primary care provider
5. Comprehensive, holistic focus on each patient's needs
6. Active engagement of patients and caregivers, including education and support
7. Emphasis on early identification and response to health care risks and symptoms to minimize complications and reduce readmissions

8. Multidisciplinary approach that includes the patient, family, and informal and formal caregivers as part of a team
9. Physician-nurse collaboration
10. Communication to, between, and among the patient, family, caregivers, and health care providers

Transitions of Care Checklist

The National Transitions of Care Coalition (NTOCC) has developed a Transitions of Care Checklist to help organizations improve communication during transitions of care (*see* Figure 4-6, pages 40–43). The checklist outlines four overarching concepts for transitions of care[4]:

1. Engagement
2. Collaboration
3. Strength-based assessment
4. Assessment as an ongoing process

The checklist also outlines common elements for assessment and intervention[4]:

- Physiological functioning
- Psychosocial functioning
- Cultural factors
- Health literacy and linguistic factors
- Financial factors
- Spiritual and religious functioning
- Physical and environmental safety
- Family and community support
- Assessment of medical issues
- Continuity/coordination of care communication

Standard Operating Protocol for Bedside Handover

Conducting transitions of care at the bedside has become common practice in many organizations. Transitions of care at the bedside allow for patient and family participation in the patient's care. Based on research conducted on six wards in two hospitals in Queensland and Western Australia that demonstrated that bedside handovers (transitions of care at the bedside) were a successful means of communication in a variety of clinical settings, Griffith University, Australia, developed a standard operating protocol for bedside handover[5] (see Figure 4-7, page 44, for an overview of the process for nurses).

Standard Operating Protocol for Whiteboard Communication

Whiteboard communication has been used for many years for communication between nurses and between nurses and ancillary personnel. Based on research conducted on four

Table 4-1. Examples for Using the SBAR Technique

Scenario Example	Descriptions	Using the SBAR Technique
1.	Mr. Jones, on med/surg unit, with history of spontaneous pneumo-thorax in past. He was admitted two days ago for pneumonia, doing well on 2L of O_2 with 95% saturation. The patient acutely developed worsening shortness of breath with decreasing O_2 sats to 85% on 100% non-rebreather mask and distress. Physical exam revealed decreased breath sounds on the right with tracheal shift.	**S**ituation: "Mr. Jones in Room 206 is in increased respiratory distress." **B**ackground: "He was admitted two days ago, history of spontaneous pneumothorax, O_2 saturation has dropped from 95% on two liters/min to 85% on non-rebreather. Auscultated his breath sounds, decreased on right, tracheal shift, increasing distress." **A**ssessment: "I am concerned he has a tension pneumo." **R**ecommendation: "Please come down right away—he may need a chest tube."
2.	The patient is in the operating room being prepped by the anesthesiologist for an interscalene block on the left side; however, the nurse knows that the patient is scheduled for right-sided shoulder surgery.	**S**ituation: "Dr. Smith, I need a little CLARITY here regarding the correct surgical side." **B**ackground: "The schedule says the operative site is on the RIGHT, and we're all set to do the block, but on the LEFT side." **A**ssessment: "I'm concerned that we may be on the WRONG side." **R**ecommendation: "We need to take a minute and make sure we've got this right. Let's re-check the schedule and the consent form. If there's any question, I recommend we get the orthopedic surgeons in here to clarify before we go any further. Agree?"
3.	Toward the end of an operative case, the circulating nurse identifies that the sponge count is off, despite looking throughout the room and counting three times. The anesthesiologist is preparing to wake the patient.	**S**ituation: "Dr. Preston, our sponge count is wrong." **B**ackground: "I know you are getting ready to wake up the patient, but we have looked extensively and counted three times, and we're still off." **A**ssessment: "I don't know if there's anything in the patient, but we have to be sure." **R**ecommendation: "I recommend we keep the patient asleep until we can shoot an x-ray and look at it."

Figure 4-6. Transitions of Care Checklist

This checklist can help improve communication between providers.

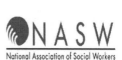

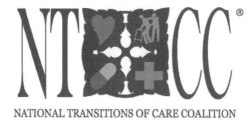

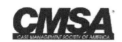

NATIONAL TRANSITIONS OF CARE COALITION

APPENDIX C
Elements of Excellence in Transitions of Care (TOC)

TOC Checklist

*The purpose of this checklist is to enhance communication—among health care providers, between care settings, and between clinicians and clients/caregivers—of patient assessments, care plans, and other essential clinical information. The checklist can serve as an adjunct to each provider's assessment tool, reinforcing the need to communicate patient care information during transitions of care. This list may also identify areas that providers do not currently assess but may wish to incorporate in the patient's record. Every element on this checklist may not be relevant to each provider or setting.

*For purposes of brevity, the term *patient/client* is used throughout this checklist to describe the client and client system (or patient and family). The *patient/client system* (or family), as defined by each patient/client, may include biological relatives, spouses or partners, friends, neighbors, colleagues, and other members of the patient/client's informal support network. Depending on the setting in which this checklist is used, providers may wish to substitute *resident, consumer, beneficiary, individual*, or other terms for *patient/client*.

Overarching Concepts

Engagement
- Maximize patient/client involvement in all phases of intervention by promoting self-determination and informed decision-making.
- Provide educational information to support the patient/client's participation in the plan of care.
- Protect patient/client's right to privacy and safeguard confidentiality when releasing patient/client information.
- Affirm patient/client dignity and respect cultural, religious, socioeconomic, and sexual diversity.
- Assess and promote the patient/client's efforts to participate in the plan of care.

(continued on page 41)

Figure 4-6. Transitions of Care Checklist, *continued*

Collaboration
- Define multidisciplinary team participants.
- Build relationships with all team members, with the patient/client at the center of the collaborative model.
- Communicate with other professionals and organizations, delineating respective responsibilities.
- Create awareness of patient/client and provider accountability for receiving and sending patient/client care information to and from care settings.
- Provide services within the bounds of professional competency and refer patient/client as needed.

Strengths-based assessment
- Use respect and empathy in patient/client interactions.
- Recognize patient/client's strengths and use those abilities to effect change.
- Help patient/client use effective coping skills and insights to manage current crises.
- Recognize and help resolve patient/client's difficulties.
- Distinguish cultural norms and behaviors from challenging behaviors.

Assessment as an ongoing process
- Keep assessments flexible, varying with presenting problem or opportunity.
- Regularly reassess patient/client's needs and progress in meeting objectives.
- Facilitate goal-setting discussion based upon the patient/client's needs during all phases of care.
- Assess effectiveness of interventions in achieving patient/client's goals.
- Communicate changes in assessment and care plan to the health care team.

Common Elements for Assessment and Intervention

Physiological functioning
- Assess patient/client's understanding of diagnosis, treatment options, and prognosis.
- Evaluate patient/client's life care planning and advance directive status.
- Evaluate impact of illness, injury, or treatments on physical, psychosocial, and sexual functioning.
- Evaluate patient/client's ability to return to or exceed pre-illness or pre-injury function level.

Psychosocial functioning
- Assess past and current mental health, emotional, cognitive, social, behavioral, or substance use/abuse concerns that may affect adjustment to illness and care management needs.
- Assess effect of medical illness or injury on psychological, emotional, cognitive, behavioral, and social functioning.

(continued on page 42)

Figure 4-6. Transitions of Care Checklist, *continued*

- Determine with patient/client which psychosocial services are needed to maximize coping.

Cultural factors
- Affirm patient/client dignity and respect cultural, religious, socioeconomic, and sexual diversity.
- Assess cultural values and beliefs, including perceptions of illness, disability, and death.
- Use the patient/client's values and beliefs to strengthen the support system.
- Understand traditions and values of patient/client groups as they relate to health care and decision-making.

Health literacy and linguistic factors
- Provide information and services in patient/client's preferred language, using translation services and interpreters.
- Use effective tools to measure patient/client's health literacy.
- Provide easy-to-understand, clinically appropriate material in layperson's language.
- Use graphic representations for patients/clients with limited language proficiency or literacy.
- Check to ensure accurate communication using teach-back methods.
- Develop educational plan based upon patient/client's identified needs.
- Evaluate caregiver's capacity to understand and apply health care information in assisting patient/client.

Financial factors
- Identify patient/client's access to, type of, and ability to navigate health insurance.
- Identify patient/client's access to and ability to navigate prescription benefits.
- Evaluate impact of illness on financial resources and ability to earn a living wage.
- Provide feedback on financial impact of treatment options.
- Educate patient/client about benefit options and how to access available resources.
- Assess barriers to accessing care and identify solutions to ensure access.

Spiritual and religious functioning
- Assess how patient/client finds meaning in life.
- Assess how spirituality and religion affect adaptation to illness.

Physical and environmental safety
- Evaluate patient/client's ability to perform activities of daily living and meet basic needs.
- Assess environmental barriers that may compromise the patient/client's ability to meet established treatment goals.
- Determine with patient/client the appropriate level of care.
- Assess ability of family or other informal caregivers to assist patient/client.

(continued on page 43)

Figure 4-6. Transitions of Care Checklist, *continued*

- Assess for risk of harm to self or others.

Family and community support
- Identify patient/client's formal and informal support systems.
- Assess how patient/client's illness affects family structure and roles.
- Provide support to family members and other informal caregivers.
- Assess for, and if appropriate help resolve, conflicts within the family.
- Evaluate risk of physical, emotional, or financial abuse or neglect, referring to community social services as needed.

Assessment of medical issues
- Patient/client diagnosis
- Symptoms
- Medication list and reconciliation of new medications throughout treatment
- Adherence assessment and intention
- Substance use and abuse disorders
- Lab tests, consultations, x-rays, and other relevant test results

Continuity/Coordination or Care Communication
- Specific clinical providers
- Date information sent to referring physician, PCP, or other clinical providers
- Necessary follow-up care

Example of Assessment & Coordination of Care Communication Checklist & Tool

Medication Assessment:
- ☑ Review all prescribed medications, over-the-counter medications, and health/nutritional supplements

Name of Medication
Dose
Route
Frequency
Next Refill

Can the patient/client tell you:
  Reason she or he is taking medication
  Positive effects of taking medication
  Symptoms or side effects of taking medication
  Where the medication is kept at home
  The next refill date for the medication
  How long she or he needs to remain on the medication

Source: National Transitions of Care Coalition: *Elements of Excellence in Transitions of Care (TOC): TOC Checklist.* http://www.ntocc.org/Portals/0/TOC_Checklist.pdf (accessed Aug. 22, 2010). Used with permission.

Figure 4-7. Overview of Bedside Nursing Handover

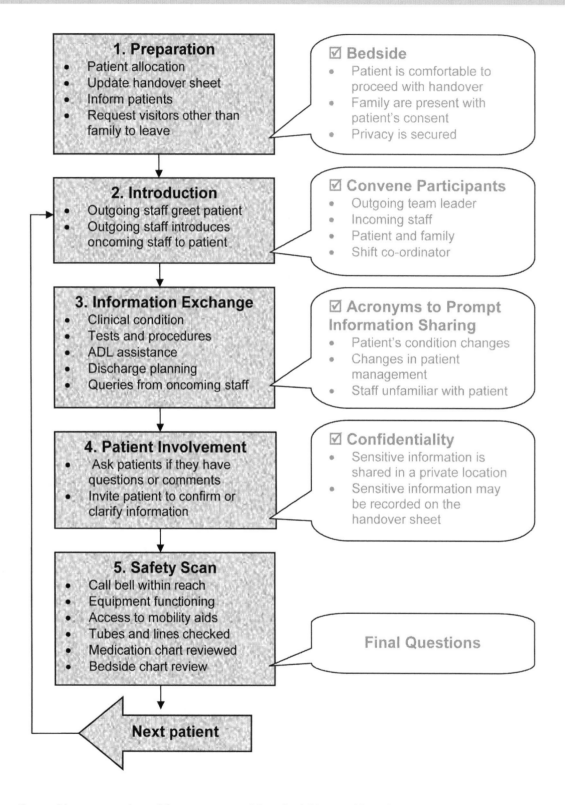

1. Preparation
- Patient allocation
- Update handover sheet
- Inform patients
- Request visitors other than family to leave

☑ **Bedside**
- Patient is comfortable to proceed with handover
- Family are present with patient's consent
- Privacy is secured

2. Introduction
- Outgoing staff greet patient
- Outgoing staff introduces oncoming staff to patient

☑ **Convene Participants**
- Outgoing team leader
- Incoming staff
- Patient and family
- Shift co-ordinator

3. Information Exchange
- Clinical condition
- Tests and procedures
- ADL assistance
- Discharge planning
- Queries from oncoming staff

☑ **Acronyms to Prompt Information Sharing**
- Patient's condition changes
- Changes in patient management
- Staff unfamiliar with patient

4. Patient Involvement
- Ask patients if they have questions or comments
- Invite patient to confirm or clarify information

☑ **Confidentiality**
- Sensitive information is shared in a private location
- Sensitive information may be recorded on the handover sheet

5. Safety Scan
- Call bell within reach
- Equipment functioning
- Access to mobility aids
- Tubes and lines checked
- Medication chart reviewed
- Bedside chart review

Final Questions

Next patient

This schematic provides an overview of the process used for a bedside transition of care.

Source: Griffith University, Australia. Used with permission.

different wards of the same hospital that demonstrated that whiteboards can be a successful means of communication for multidisciplinary teams, Griffith University, Australia, developed a standard operating protocol for whiteboard communication[6] (*see* Figure 4-8, page 46, for an overview of the process).

Use of Technology to Streamline Transition Processes

Computerized systems allow for the transfer of valuable, up-to-date clinical information without the need for interruptions in work flow. When systems are integrated into the electronic health record or electronic medical record, patient information becomes easily accessible to providers throughout the organization (*see* Sidebar 4-2, page 47). Other benefits of using technology for transitions of care include the following[7,8]:

• Information can be readily and easily updated.
• Information can be accessed from many locations, including home.
• It can enhance morale due to better communication between nurses and physicians.
• It allows for easy identification of the patient's physician.
• Current problems and solutions are easily communicated.

Electronic systems that allow for the transfer of information across settings and between care providers help with continuity and coordination of care. For example, automated medication reconciliation between care settings, such as physician's offices and the hospital, streamlines and increases safety during admissions and discharges.[8]

The University of Washington, Seattle, developed a Web-based resident sign-out system that draws information from the patient's electronic medical record and also allows residents to enter data.[9] The University of Washington Computerized Rounding and Sign-Out System (UWCores) is available through any secure Internet connection. "UWCores does not replace a conversation between primary and cross-covering or night float providers," says Erik Van Eaton, M.D., who was a surgery resident at the University of Washington, Seattle, when the program was developed. "We still believe that conversation is required and can accommodate the majority of question-and-answer communication. However, UWCores ensures that for each patient, a 'minimum data set' is transferred to the oncoming clinician, even if that information is never conveyed during an actual conversation between providers."[9]

The UWCores system was built around resident work flow. "There are a lot of reservations among some groups as to how electronic systems will fit in with their work flow," Van Eaton says. "That's why it's important to build these systems around that work flow, so you can diminish that up-front resistance. In the case of UWCores, the residents knew it would make their jobs easier, so they were desperate to use it."[9]

As reported in July 2010, an intervention has been created at Brigham and Women's Hospital in Boston "that automatically triggers an e-mail with the finalized test results to the responsible providers." Anuj Dalal, M.D. explains, "The intervention creates a loop of communication between the inpatient attending [physician] and the PCP [primary care physician]. What we hope to show in our research over the next year or two is whether the intervention actually increases awareness of test results by providers."[10]

Another technological tool, in pilot testing in 2010, is an application designed for mobile "smart phones" that would allow real-time messaging and the systematic transfer of key information from one hospitalist to another at shift changes. Vineet Chopra, M.D., a hospitalist at the University of Michigan Health System in Ann Arbor who has been working on the development of the application, emphasizes that the goal in developing any new technology is to make "life easier" for those who will actually use it. "I'm not a believer in throwing more technology at problems and just adding more layers of information tools [that have no practical benefit]," he says. He also cautions that technology is not a substitute for "the face-to-face encounter that needs to happen" between providers and patients.[10]

Solutions That Work in Paper-to-Technology Types of Transitions

Organizations that use technology such as electronic health records might find transitions of care challenging when a patient enters the organization from a paper-based facility (for example, coming from a physician's office to a hospital). This transition can be particularly difficult if documents come in from multiple locations—such as a long term care facility, the patient's family physician, and the patient's pharmacy—and need to be scanned to the patient's chart.

The following strategies can help organizations better maintain complete and accurate medical records during paper-to-technology transitions[11]:

• Take the time to review all information in the patient's record. Review the patient's history and physical

Figure 4-8. Overview of Whiteboard Communication in Medium-Stay Medical Units

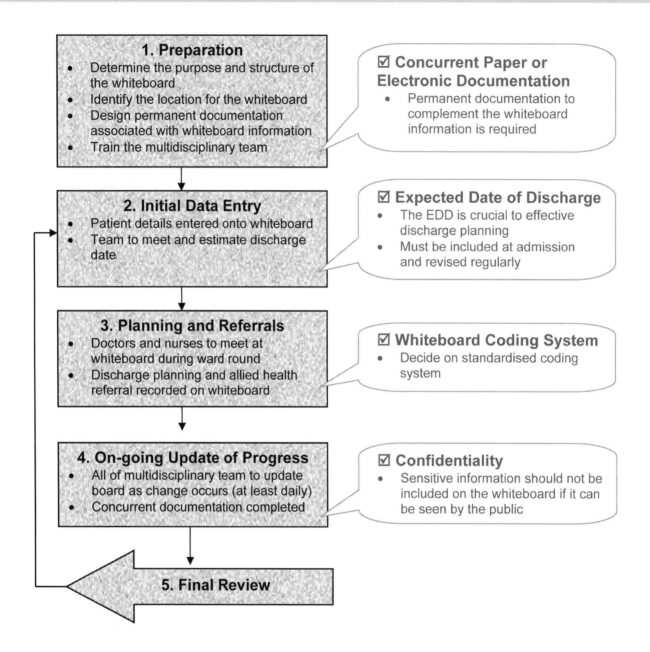

This schematic provides an overview of the whiteboard communication process on medium-stay medical units.

Source: Griffith University, Australia. Used with permission.

Sidebar 4-2. Benefits of Electronic Health Records

An electronic health record is more than just an electronic version of a patient's paper medical file. It includes key administrative clinical data pertinent to the patient's care under a particular provider. Such data as demographics, past medical history, progress notes, prescription records, vital signs, immunizations, test results and laboratory data, and radiology reports all can be found in an electronic health record.

In an ideal situation, the electronic health record in a physician's office will interface with the radiology department, the pharmacy, and the hospital, providing seamless care to the patient and a faster work flow for the provider.

Physicians who have important patient information at their fingertips (such as allergies, family history, and current prescription drugs) are able to make better decisions about the care they provide. For example, knowing a patient's complete list of current prescription medications may alert the physician to possible drug interactions before a new medication is prescribed. Familiarity with a patient's family history could alert the physician that further tests are needed. Having a complete electronic file of radiology and lab reports allows a physician to review the patient's history and avoid ordering duplicate tests, thereby saving both time and money.

Electronic health records incorporate decision-making technology and tools based on evidence-based medicine and other comprehensive information. This point-of-care decision support assists physicians in evaluating and tracking treatment protocols, and it enables them to diagnose and treat serious illnesses more immediately and effectively. Additionally, the instant connection to evidence-based clinical guidelines can help increase preventive care support services and improve the overall management of chronic disease.

Many electronic health records allow providers access to computerized order entry systems (also known as computerized provider order entry [CPOE] systems), which may result in better formulary compliance, clearer prescriptions (which decreases pharmacy call-backs), and simplification of medication refills.

Another benefit of electronic health records is that they allow for monitoring of patient safety issues or initiatives. For example, they may be used to monitor incidents of patient falls or medication errors so that negative trends may be more easily detected and corrected.

On a global level, many health care professionals believe that storing health information electronically will lead to greater communication both within organizations and across health care institutions and agencies. For example, electronic health records could be used to provide a global database for medical research or to assist with the recognition of public health threats.

information, along with all the assessments, and then go back to the plan of care. There should be consistency between the assessments, the plan of care, and the documentation that supports the plan of care.

- Provide feedback to individuals when documentation is lacking. If a particular facility consistently omits important patient information, such as diagnostic test results, contact that facility and ask that the facility include that information when its patients or residents are admitted.
- Provide staff with examples of good processes that are related to specific documentation problem areas. For example, a good process for ensuring that paper-based records are entered into the electronic medical record might be an electronic checklist to compare the documents that are needed to those that have actually been received and scanned.
- Use the "Plan, Do, Study, Act" method of developing standardized methods for collecting and entering paper-based documents into the electronic medical record (that is, develop a plan, execute, evaluate, and make adjustments if necessary). Also, involve the people who will be doing the collection and entry in the development of related policies.

Many organizations around the world have successfully made the transition from paper records to electronic health records. The following are examples of organizations that have successfully implemented an electronic health record system.

Institute for Quality at DeKalb Medical Center, Decatur and Hillansdale, Georgia

Using a benefits scorecard to measure the impact of electronic health record implementation, the Institute for Quality at DeKalb Medical Center—a U.S. health care organization with facilities in Decatur and Hillansdale, Georgia—tracked the baseline data before implementation and change related to electronic health record adoption. The electronic health record was configured to support computerized provider order entry, evidence-based order sets, and automated medication dosing. The Institute for Quality reported that adoption of the electronic health record led to the following results:

- A 66% reduction in medication administration–related errors, including wrong medication, wrong patient, and wrong route
- An 89% reduction in medication-related errors, such as errors of omission and duplicate medication orders
- An 80% reduction in errors connected to delayed medication administration

Health First, Rockledge, Florida

After implementing an electronic health record system to conduct a system-enabled redesign of its surgical work flows, including registration, preadmission testing, preoperative services, operating room, and postanesthesia care unit, the U.S. health care organization Health First in Rockledge, Florida, experienced better quality and efficiency in all processes.

With the electronic health record system, Health First reported an increased consistency in medication documentation and eliminated unapproved abbreviations and transcription errors at all hospitals. At one medical center, the documentation quality of surgical infection prevention protocols reportedly improved by 64% in a 4-month period. At all sites, the electronic health record supported creating care plans and building scripts to streamline correct and complete documentation.

Wan Fang Hospital, Taipei, Taiwan

Wan Fang Hospital is a large medical center in Taipei, Taiwan. Students at Taipei Medical University who are training to become physicians and surgeons serve their internships at Wan Fang Hospital. Following the implementation of a computerized provider order entry system at Wan Fang Hospital in January 2007, the adverse medication event rate of near misses among inpatients reportedly was reduced from 2.19% to 0.25%.

Al Ain Hospital, United Arab Emirates

Al Ain Hospital in Al Ain, United Arab Emirates, recently introduced an electronic health record system to improve hospital business functions and eventually eliminate paper medical records. The hospital's immediate goals were to improve patient safety, enhance patient confidentiality, and reduce the need for additional testing.

The implementation of the new application was to be deployed in phases. The first phase was successfully launched on November 5, 2009. It involved the facility's outpatient clinics, emergency department, and all hospital departments. The electronic health record system improved several functions within Al Ain Hospital, such as registration, scheduling, medical records, radiology, outpatient pharmacies, and physician order entry. The planned second phase for 2010 was to include additional clinical functionality and cover the pharmacy and clinical notes.

National Skin Centre, Singapore

The National Skin Centre, an outpatient facility in Singapore specializing in dermatology, in 2000 implemented a fully integrated electronic health record system designed specifically for its own needs. Senior medical, nursing, operations, pharmacy, and laboratory personnel were involved in the implementation process, which was deployed for the entire center simultaneously.

Careful consideration was given to patient safety issues, including patient identification, privacy and confidentiality issues, security, and drug allergy issues. Patient safety features of the National Skin Centre's electronic health record system include the following:
• Drug allergy alert
• High-alert medication
• Monitoring of lab results
• Abnormal lab results alert
• Reduced prescription error with e-orders
• Methicillan-resistant *Staphylococcus aureus* alert
• Fall risk patient alert

Medication Reconciliation Policies and Procedures

Medication reconciliation can be difficult when no standardized process exists to collect medication information and ensure that it is available to care providers. It is helpful to have standardized processes in place for the following[12]:
• Compiling a complete, current, and accurate medication list
• Conducting a medication reconciliation of that list
• Initiating new medication orders and updating the medication list
• Communicating the current list to the patient and the next provider of care

Some organizations may already have standardized processes but may find that they are not as effective as they had hoped. In other organizations, staff from different units, or within the same unit, may be using different processes for medication reconciliation. Regardless of the processes an organization has employed, physicians need a defined method for communicating changes in medication orders. Figure 4-9, page 50, shows four basic steps that could be standardized in any medication reconciliation process.

The following elements are useful to include in all medication reconciliation policies and procedures:
• A clear definition of medication reconciliation
• A list of types of medications to be considered in the reconciliation process
• A description of each discipline's responsibilities in the medication reconciliation process

• Steps for comparing the patient's preadmission medications with medications prescribed by the organization
• Paper or electronic forms to be used

Compiling the Medication List

Compiling the medication list (collecting an accurate and complete record of all medications the patient was taking before entering the health care system) may be the most difficult part of the medication reconciliation process.

The medication list ideally would include the following[13,14]:
• Patient allergies
• Prescription medications (listing product name, dosage, route, frequency, time of last dose, and reason for use), including samples
• Over-the-counter products taken by the patient, including herbals, vitamins, dietary supplements, homeopathic products, home remedies, and nutraceuticals
• Other therapies, such as respiratory therapy products, parenteral nutrition, blood derivatives, and intravenous solutions
• Less-common therapies, which may include recently administered vaccines, diagnostic and contrast agents, or radioactive medications

A sample form for recording medications is provided in Figure 4-10, page 51.

Creating an accurate medication list may require the use of multiple resources, including the patient or caregiver, historical records, the patient's pharmacist, the patient's primary care physician, and the patient's medication bottles. Each of these resources has the following benefits and limitations:
• The patient or caregiver is in the best position to know what medications the patient is taking but may not always know the dosage. Patients and caregivers also may forget to report over-the-counter (nonprescription) medications.
• Historical records can provide detailed information but may not always be accurate.
• The patient's pharmacist may be a good initial source of information, but pharmacy medication profiles may only include prescription medications, and the pharmacist has no way of knowing whether the patient is complying with dosage instructions. Many patients use multiple pharmacies, which increases the possibility that medications may be missed if only the primary pharmacy is contacted.
• The patient's primary care provider also is a good initial source of information, but primary care providers may not

Figure 4-9. Basic Steps of Medication Reconciliation

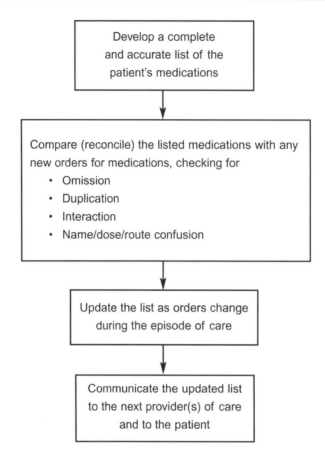

This basic flowchart identifies four fundamental steps that could be standardized in the medication reconciliation process.

Source: Richard J. Croteau, M.D., patient safety advisor, Joint Commission International.

always be informed when their patients are given a prescription by another specialist.

- Medication bottles are a good source of information because they provide not only the medication names but also the dosages. However, patients may not be following the dosage instructions and may not remember to bring over-the-counter products when providing caregivers with medication bottles.

When the patient's medication list cannot be acquired through any of the usual channels, external sources such as community hospitals, long term care facilities, rehabilitation and step-down facilities, home care agencies, and organized health plans may be able to provide information about the patient's medications.

Reconciling Medications with New Orders

After the patient's medication list has been compiled, it needs to be compared against new orders that are written during admission, transfer, and discharge. Prescribers should have access to a complete and current medication list at all times during the patient's stay. A sample physician admission and discharge medication reconciliation form is provided in Figure 4-11, page 52.

Because reconciliation of the patient's medication list with new orders requires knowledge of medications and their potential to interact with other medications, the pharmacist typically performs the actual reconciliation, particularly on admission. However, in some organizations, reconciliation is the responsibility of the physician or an advance practice nurse.

Figure 4-10. General Medication Reconciliation Form

TITLE: **ADMISSION MEDICATION LIST/ORDER**							Page _____ of _____		

NOTE: ❑ THESE ORDERS CAN BE CHECKED BY THE PHYSICIAN TO DESIGNATE FURTHER INSTRUCTIONS.

DO NOT USE THE FOLLOWING ABBREVIATIONS: U or u; Q.D., QD, q.d., qd; Q.O.D. QOD, qod, q.o.d., IU, MS or MSO4 or MgSO4; trailing zero; lack of leading zero

Allergies/Reaction _____
_____ ❑ Anesthesia ❑ Blood ❑ Food ❑ Latex

Height _____ Weight _____ Could you be pregnant: ❑ Yes ❑ No ❑ N/A Lactating: ❑ Yes ❑ No ❑ N/A
Source of medication history: ❑ patient ❑ family ❑ pharmacy ❑ ECF
❑ Rx bottles ❑ past admission ❑ other _____ ❑ No medications taken at home
MEDICATIONS PRIOR TO ADMISSION *(Includes prescription over the counter, herbal products, and supplements)*

Continued Admission Yes / No	Drug Name (List only currently being taken)	Dose (mg, ml, number, gms)	Route/ Topical Site	Frequency (How often)	Date/Time of Last Dose	DISCHARGE MEDICATIONS	
						Resume at same dose	DO NOT Resume at Discharge
❑ ❑	1.					❑	❑
❑ ❑	2.					❑	❑
❑ ❑	3.					❑	❑
❑ ❑	4.					❑	❑
❑ ❑	5.					❑	❑
❑ ❑	6.					❑	❑
❑ ❑	7.					❑	❑
❑ ❑	8.					❑	❑
❑ ❑	9.					❑	❑
❑ ❑	10.					❑	❑
❑ ❑	11.					❑	❑
❑ ❑	12.					❑	❑
❑ ❑	13.					❑	❑
❑ ❑	14.					❑	❑
❑ ❑	15.					❑	❑
❑ ❑	16.					❑	❑
❑ ❑	17.					❑	❑

Signature of person completing form _____ Date _____ Time _____

Admission Physician Signature _____ Date _____ Time _____

Discharge Physician Signature _____ Date _____ Time _____

D T 0 2 7 9

Mount Carmel, Columbus, Ohio
Admission Medication List/Order
45250-10-08

NAME

DOB

MR #

FAN #

This form can be used to record a complete list of a patient's medications. The form shown here also has boxes for the provider to mark to indicate which medications should be resumed after discharge.

Source: Mount Carmel East Hospital, Columbus, Ohio. Used with permission.

Figure 4-11. Physician Admission and Discharge Medication Reconciliation Form

Miami Valley Hospital
Dayton, Ohio

PHYSICIAN ADMISSION & DISCHARGE MEDICATION ORDERS

Height	Weight
	est act kg

Keep this form in green plastic folder in front of Physician Orders

Allergies □ Contrast media □ Latex
□ Food □ Adhesive tape □ Shellfish
□ Iodine

□ Pregnant   □ Breast Feeding   □ N/A

Source of medication list:
□ Pt/Family recall   □ Pt medication list   □ MAR from facility
□ PCP List   □ List copied and placed   □ Medications brought
□ Previous d/c paperwork   in chart   from home

Pharmacy (Name/Phone No.)

Discharge Medications

"Home" Prescription & Over the Counter Medications		Product Name (List those currently being taken)	Dose (mg, ml, number & gms)	Route or Topical Site	Frequency	Date & Time of Last Dose	Resume at same dose	DO NOT Resume at discharge
Order								
□ Yes □ No	□ Already ordered						□	□
□ Yes □ No	□ Already ordered						□	□
□ Yes □ No	□ Already ordered						□	□
□ Yes □ No	□ Already ordered						□	□
□ Yes □ No	□ Already ordered						□	□
□ Yes □ No	□ Already ordered						□	□
□ Yes □ No	□ Already ordered						□	□
□ Yes □ No	□ Already ordered						□	□
□ Yes □ No	□ Already ordered						□	□
□ Yes □ No	□ Already ordered						□	□
□ Yes □ No	□ Already ordered						□	□

Herbal Products NOT TO BE TAKEN IN HOSPITAL (Herbals will <u>not</u> be dispensed by MVH Pharmacy)

Discharge Disposition

□ Home
□ Home Health Care
□ ECF - See ECF packet for med list

□ Outpatient therapy
   □ PT □ OT □ Corp
   □ Speech
   □ Other _____

□ Instruct Patient to take only those medications ordered at discharge until instructed otherwise

Date/Time _____ RN Obtaining Medication History Signature _____

Physician Signature _____ Date/Time _____ HUC Signature _____ Date/Time _____

Physician Printed Name _____ Date/Time _____ RN/LPN Signature _____ Date/Time _____

ADDITIONAL DISCHARGE MEDICATION ORDERS

Product Name	Dose	Frequency	Route or Topical Site	Script
				□
				□
				□
				□
				□

Physician Signature _____ Date/Time _____

Physician Printed Name _____ Date/Time _____

F/U Appt: _____
□ D/C Foley   □ D/C IV Access   □ PICC line care @ home
□ Dressing changes or treatments
Activities: □ Resume usual activity   □ Limited activity
Diet: □ Regular   □ Low fat   □ Low sodium   □ ADA   □ Other _____
Other:

PHO-6006 (6/2006)

Staff members use this order sheet to reconcile medications at admission and discharge, and the prescriber indicates orders with the same form.

Source: Miami Valley Hospital, Dayton, Ohio. Rodehaver C., Fearing D.: Medication reconciliation in acute care: Ensuring an accurate drug regimen on admission and discharge. *Jt Comm J Qual Patient Saf* 31:406–413, Jul. 2005.

Communicating the List at Discharge or Transfer

When a patient is discharged or transferred to another setting, service, provider, level of care, or facility, it is important that a complete list of the patient's current medications be communicated to the next provider or facility. Reconciling medications as patients are discharged or transferred provides a means to check medication orders and helps prevent medication errors. Any discrepancies can be brought to the prescriber's attention, and, if appropriate, changes can be made.

It is helpful to utilize a standardized form or template to communicate medication information during transfer or discharge. A standardized form can be used to do the following[13]:

- Document medications ordered on transfer or discharge for the medical record
- Provide information on how to obtain clarification of unclear orders or prescriptions
- Act as a prescription to be filled by an outside pharmacy
- Provide an external transfer summary and communicate an accurate list of patient medications for another unit or institution
- Supply patient medication instructions

Contingency Planning

It may not always be possible to reach prescribers to clarify orders or inform them of medication discrepancies. It is useful for organizations to develop policies for when to contact the prescriber at home and for appropriate utilization of other qualified individuals to make clinical decisions when the prescriber is unavailable.

Because health care organizations are busy places, there will be times when high patient volume or staffing shortages can interfere with the medication reconciliation process. It is helpful to develop contingency plans that include cross-training of additional staff to perform medication reconciliation functions.

Educating Patients About Medications at Discharge

When a patient is being discharged, it is extremely helpful for organizations to provide a list of current medications to both the patient and the patient's primary care provider (*see* Figure 4-12, page 54). A discharge discussion provides an excellent opportunity for the provider to educate patients and their caregivers about the patients' medications and about the importance of maintaining the medication list.

Before the patient is discharged from the facility, it is useful to emphasize any changes in the medications that the patient was taking prior to admission and to review new medications again. Give the patient instructions regarding how and for how long to continue taking any newly prescribed medications. Patients who have been well educated about follow-up care are more likely to recover more quickly and less likely to require readmission.

Patient Education Tool: Help Avoid Mistakes with Your Medicine

As part of its Speak Up™ campaign (*see* Sidebar 4-3, page 55), The Joint Commission developed a brochure to help caregivers educate patients about avoiding medication errors. The brochure includes answers to frequently asked questions about medications, what patients should know about their medications, what they should do if they miss a dose, how patients can help avoid medication errors, and what to ask the physician or pharmacist. It also includes a medication list. The brochure is available in English and Spanish (*see* Figures 4-13 and 4-14, pages 56–57 and 58–59, respectively).

Ways to Address Health Literacy Issues

It is sometimes difficult for caregivers to know which patients have low health literacy skills. Although people with low health literacy skills tend to be poor, less educated, and elderly, and may have physical and mental disabilities, demographic information alone is not a reliable indicator of a person's health literacy.

Staff members need to be taught to recognize the behaviors of patients with low health literacy skills, which may not be easy because many patients have become adept at hiding their deficiencies. The following behaviors may indicate a literacy problem[15,16]:

- Avoiding situations that require reading
- Claiming to have left reading glasses at home
- Complaining of headaches or other health problems too severe to allow reading
- Asking to bring written documents home to discuss with a spouse or child
- Not asking questions
- Being unable to restate information in own words
- Supplying incomplete or inaccurate registration forms
- Not complying with medication regimens
- Frequently missing appointments
- Failing to schedule or missing appointments for laboratory tests, imaging tests, or referrals to subspecialists

Figure 4-12. Sample Home Medication List

MCG Health, Inc.
Medication Reconciliation -- Home Medication List
Today's date _____

Name |_____|

DOB or MRN |_____|

Admission

Date, Interviewer Initials	List all medications to which patient is allergic:	How severe is the reaction?				
		Severe	Moderate	Mild	Unknown	Reaction
	☐ No Known Drug Allergies					

List all medications including prescription, over-the-counter, herbals or "natural remedies" and periodic in-office injections

Date, Interviewer Initials	Medication	Dosage	How often?	Reason Taken (optional)	Continue as Inpatient? (check)
					☐Yes☐No
					☐Yes☐No
					☐Yes☐No
					☐Yes☐No
					☐Yes☐No
					☐Yes☐No
					☐Yes☐No
					☐Yes☐No
					☐Yes☐No
					☐Yes☐No
					☐Yes☐No
					☐Yes☐No
					☐Yes☐No
					☐Yes☐No
					☐Yes☐No
					☐Yes☐No
					☐Yes☐No

☐ Does not currently take any medications. Reviewed med list with patient and/or family ☐Yes ☐No
Verified med list against medication bottle labels?? ☐Yes ☐No

Comments (including any updates):

Signature/Title /Initials/Date

_____   _____

_____   _____

This is not an order. To be filed as the first page in the Orders section as a reference for admission and discharge medication orders.

Rev. 10/13/08; FOD FORM MCG339

ORDER

A medication list, such as this one, may be sent home with the patient at discharge.

Source: MCGHealth, Inc. Used with permission.

Sidebar 4-3. The Joint Commission's Speak Up™ Campaign

In March 2002, The Joint Commission, together with the U.S. Centers for Medicare & Medicaid Services (CMS), launched Speak Up, a national campaign urging patients to help prevent health care errors by becoming active, involved, and informed participants on the health care team. The ongoing campaign includes brochures, posters, and buttons on a variety of patient safety topics. Speak Up encourages the public to do the following:

Speak up if you have questions or concerns. If you still do not understand, ask again. It is your body and you have a right to know.

Pay attention to the care you get. Always make sure you are getting the right treatments and medicines by the right health care professionals. Do not assume anything.

Educate yourself about your illness. Learn about the medical tests you get and your treatment plan.

Ask a trusted family member or friend to be your advocate (adviser or supporter).

Know what medicines you take and why you take them. Medicine errors are the most common health care mistakes.

Use a hospital, clinic, surgery center, or other type of health care organization that has been carefully checked out. For example, The Joint Commission visits hospitals in the United States to see if they are meeting The Joint Commission's quality standards. Joint Commission International (JCI) visits hospitals in other parts of the world to see if they are meeting JCI standards.

Participate in all decisions about your treatment. You are the center of the health care team.

As part of the Speak Up campaign, The Joint Commission has developed the following patient education materials:
* Help Prevent Errors in Your Care
* Help Avoid Mistakes in Your Surgery
* Information for Living Organ Donors
* Five Things You Can Do to Prevent Infection
* Help Avoid Mistakes with Your Medicines
* What You Should Know About Research Studies
* Planning Your Follow-Up Care
* Help Prevent Medical Test Mistakes
* Know Your Rights
* Understanding Your Doctors and Other Caregivers
* What You Should Know About Pain Management
* Prevent Errors in Your Child's Care
* Stay Well and Keep Others Well (a coloring book for children)
* Tips for Your Doctor's Visit

These materials are available for free downloading on The Joint Commission Web site, http://www.jointcommission.org or for purchase through the Joint Commission Resources Web site, http://www.jcrinc.com.

Figure 4-13. Help Avoid Mistakes with Your Medicines (English Version)

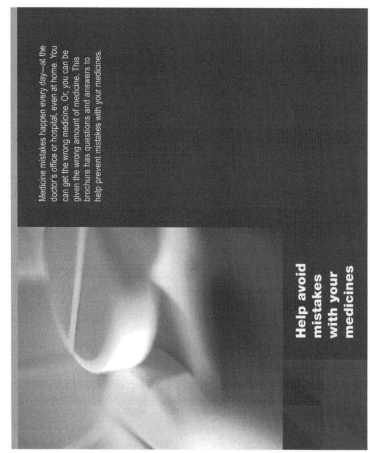

Speak**UP**™

Help avoid mistakes with your medicines

Medicine mistakes happen every day—at the doctor's office or hospital, even at home. You can get the wrong medicine. Or, you can be given the wrong amount of medicine. This brochure has questions and answers to help prevent mistakes with your medicines.

The Joint Commission

My Medicine List

Medication* (include amount you take and how often or what time of day)

vitamins

herbs, diet supplements, natural remedies

alcohol, recreational drugs

(continued on page 57)

Figure 4-13. Help Avoid Mistakes with Your Medicines (English Version), *continued*

The goal of the Speak Up™ program is to help patients become more informed and involved in their health care.

Who is responsible for your medicines?

A lot of people—including you!

- Doctors check all of your medicines to make sure they are OK to take together. They will also check your vitamins, herbs, diet supplements or natural remedies.
- Pharmacists will check your new medicines to see if there are other medicines, foods or drinks you should not take with your new medicines. This helps to avoid a bad reaction.
- Nurses and other caregivers may prepare medicines or give them to you.
- You need to give your doctors, pharmacists and other caregivers a list of your medicines. This list should have your
  - prescription medicines
  - over-the-counter medicines (for example, aspirin)
  - vitamins
  - herbs
  - diet supplements
  - natural remedies
  - amount of alcohol you drink each day or week
  - recreational drugs

This brochure has a wallet card for your list of medicines.

What should you know about your medicines?

- Make sure you can read the handwriting on the prescription. If you can't read it, the pharmacist may not be able to read it either. You can ask to have the prescription printed.
- Read the label. Make sure it has your name on it and the right medicine name.
- Make sure that you understand all of the instructions for your medicines.
- If you have doubts about a medicine, ask your doctor, pharmacist or caregiver about it.

What if you forget the instructions for taking a medicine or are not sure about taking it?

Call your doctor or pharmacist. Don't be afraid to ask questions about any of your medicines.

What can you do at the hospital or clinic to help avoid mistakes with your medicines?

- Make sure your doctors, nurses and other caregivers check your wristband and ask your name before giving you medicine. Some patients get a medicine that was supposed to go to another patient.
- Don't be afraid to tell a caregiver if you think you are about to get the wrong medicine.
- Know what time you should get a medicine. If you don't get it then, speak up.
- Tell your caregiver if you don't feel well after taking a medicine. Ask for help immediately if you think you are having a side effect or reaction.
- You may be given IV (intravenous) fluids. Read the bag to find out what is in it. Ask the caregiver how long it should take for the liquid to run out. Tell the caregiver if it's dripping too fast or too slow.
- Get a list of your medicines—including your new ones. Read the list carefully. Make sure it lists everything you are taking. If you're not well enough to do this, ask a friend or relative to help.

Questions to ask your doctor or pharmacist

- How will this new medicine help you?
- Are there other names for this medicine? For example, does it have a brand or generic name?
- Is there any written information about the medicine?
- Can you take this medicine with your allergy? Remind your doctor about your allergies and reactions you have had to medicines.
- Is it safe to take this medicine with your other medicines? Is it safe to take it with your vitamins, herbs and supplements?
- Are there any side effects of the medicine? For example, upset stomach. Who can you call if you have side effects or a bad reaction? Can they be reached 24 hours a day, seven days a week?
- Are there specific instructions for your medicines? For example, are there any foods or drinks you should avoid while taking it?
- Can you stop taking the medicine as soon as you feel better? Or do you need to take it until it's gone?
- Do you need to swallow or chew the medicine? Can you cut or crush it if you need to?
- Is it safe to drink alcohol with the medicine?

www.jointcommission.org

It's important to include this information in case of an emergency.
Carry this card with you. Share it with your pharmacist, doctor and other caregivers.

Medication* (include amount you take and how often or what time of day)

prescription _____

over-the-counter (for example, aspirin) _____

My Medicine List

Name _____

Blood Type _____

Allergies _____

Emergency Contact _____

List all of your
prescription medicines
over-the-counter medicines (for example, aspirin)
vitamins
herbs
diet supplements
natural remedies
amount of alcohol you drink each day or week
recreational drugs

This informational brochure can help English-speaking patients better understand how to avoid medication errors. The section "My Medication List" at one end may be detached and placed in the patient's wallet.

Figure 4-14. Help Avoid Mistakes with Your Medicines (Spanish Version)

¡Hable!

Cómo evitar
errores con sus
medicamentos

Los errores en los medicamentos se
producen a diario, tanto en el consultorio
como en el hospital, y a veces hasta en
casa. Puede equivocarse de medicamento.
O, puede proporcionársele la dosis
equivocada. Este folleto incluye preguntas
y respuestas para ayudarle a evitar los
errores con sus medicamentos.

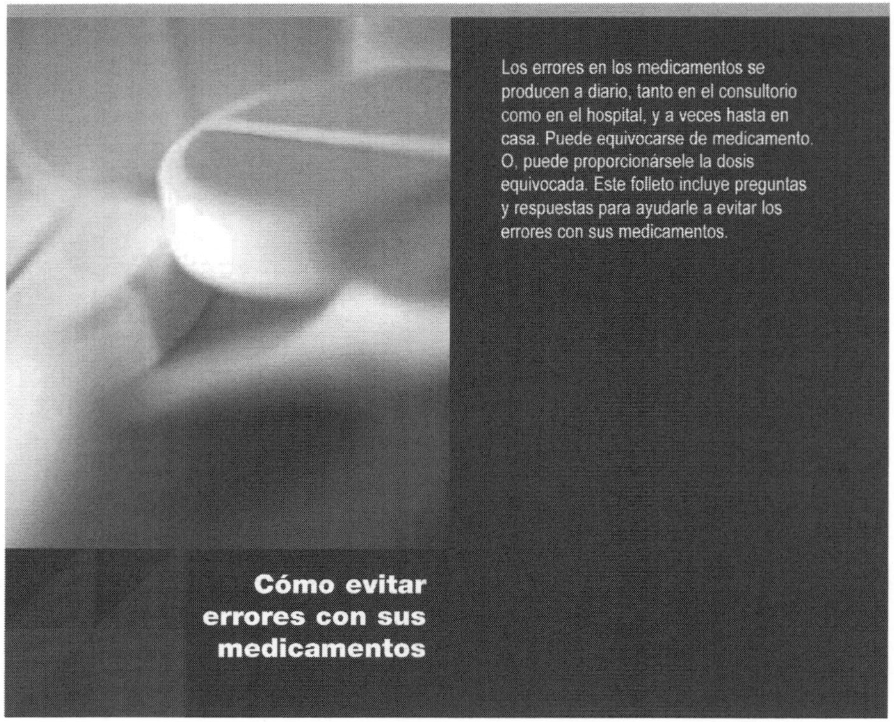

The Joint Commission

(continued on page 59)

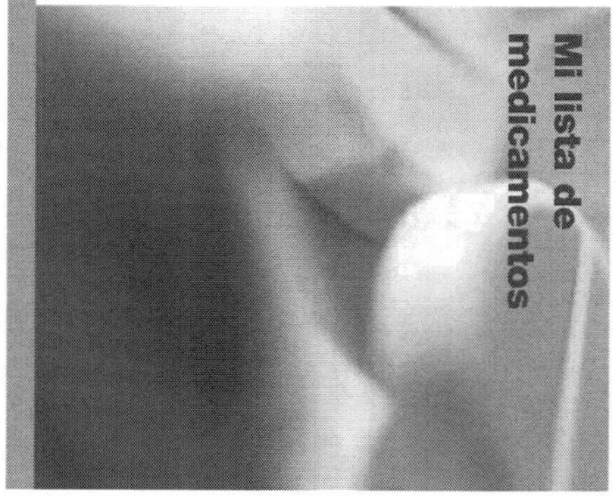

Mi lista de
medicamentos

Medicamentos (incluya la cantidad que toma y con cuánta frecuencia y a qué hora del día lo hace)

vitaminas

hierbas, complementos alimenticios, remedios naturales

alcohol, drogas recreativas

Figure 4-14. Help Avoid Mistakes with Your Medicines (Spanish Version), *continued*

El objetivo del programa "Hable" es ayudar a los pacientes a mantenerse informados y activos durante su atención médica.

¿Quién es responsable de sus medicamentos?

Mucha gente... ¡incluyéndole a usted!

- Los médicos revisan todos sus medicamentos para asegurarse de que puedan tomarse juntos. También revisan sus vitaminas, hierbas, complementos alimenticios o remedios naturales.
- Los farmacéuticos revisan sus medicamentos nuevos para ver si hay algún otro medicamento, comida o bebida que o pueda tomar con ellos. Esto le ayuda a evitar tener una mala reacción.
- Las enfermeras y otras personas que le atienden pueden preparar los medicamentos o dárselos.
- Tiene usted que darle a sus médicos, farmacéutico y a las personas que le atienden una lista de sus medicamentos. Esta lista deberá contar con todos sus
  medicamentos por prescripción
  medicamentos sin receta (por ejemplo, aspirina)
  vitaminas
  hierbas
  complementos alimenticios
  remedios naturales
  cantidad de alcohol que ingiere a diario o a la semana
  drogas recreativas

Este folleto tiene una tarjeta para que lleve en la cartera, con una lista de sus medicamentos.

¿Qué debe saber acerca de sus medicamentos por prescripción?

- Asegúrese de poder leer lo que dice la receta. Si no puede, es posible que el farmacéutico tampoco pueda. Puede pedir que le entreguen la receta impresa.
- Lea la etiqueta. Asegúrese de que tenga su nombre y de que el nombre del medicamento esté correcto. Asegúrese de que comprende todas las instrucciones de sus medicamentos.

- Si tiene cualquier duda, pregunte a su médico, farmacéutico o a la persona que le atiende.
- ¿Y si olvida las instrucciones para tomar un medicamento o no está seguro de cómo hacerlo? Llame a su médico o farmacéutico. No tema preguntar acerca de sus medicamentos.

Preguntas que debe plantear a su médico o farmacéutico

- ¿En qué le ayudará este nuevo medicamento?
- ¿Existen otros nombres para este medicamento? Por ejemplo, ¿tiene un nombre de marca y un nombre genérico?
- ¿Existe alguna información por escrito acerca de este medicamento?
- ¿Puede tomar este medicamento a pesar de su alergia? Recuerde a su médico sobre sus alergias y las reacciones que haya tenido a otros medicamentos.
- ¿Es seguro tomar este medicamento con sus otras medicinas? ¿Es seguro tomarlo con sus vitaminas, hierbas y complementos?
- ¿Tienen algún efecto secundario? Por ejemplo, revuélvele el estómago. ¿A quién puede llamar en caso de que se presenten efectos secundarios o una reacción mala? ¿Es posible localizarlos las 24 horas, los siete días de la semana?
- ¿Existen instrucciones específicas para sus medicamentos? Por ejemplo, ¿hay algún alimento o bebida que deba evitar mientras los toma?
- ¿Puede dejar de tomar el medicamento en cuanto se sienta mejor? ¿O necesita tomarlo hasta que se termine?
- ¿Es un medicamento que se traga o que se mastica? En caso necesario, ¿se puede cortar o aplastar?
- ¿Es seguro consumir alcohol cuando se toma este medicamento?

Preguntas para el hospital o la clínica

- Asegúrese de que sus médicos, enfermeras y otras personas que le atienden revisen su nombre en la pulsera y se lo pregunten antes de darle el medicamento. Algunos pacientes reciben los medicamentos que eran para otro paciente.
- No tema decirle a la persona que le atiende si cree que está a punto de recibir el medicamento equivocado.
- Sepa a qué hora debe tomar su medicamento. Si no se lo llevan, pídalo.
- Avise a quién lo cuida si no se siente bien después de tomar un medicamento. Pida ayuda de inmediato si cree que está teniendo un efecto secundario o una reacción negativa.
- Pueden proporcionársele fluidos intravenosos. Lea la bolsa para saber lo que le están poniendo. Pregunte a la persona que le atienda cuánto tiempo tardará el líquido en terminarse. Avísele si el goteo parece ser demasiado rápido o demasiado lento.
- Haga una lista de sus medicamentos, incluyendo los nuevos. Léala con atención. Asegúrese de que contiene todo lo que está usted tomando. Si no está en condiciones de hacerlo, pida ayuda a un amigo o paciente.

www.jointcommission.org

Mi lista de medicamentos

Nombre _____

Tipo de sangre _____

Alergias _____

Nombres y números telefónicos de a quién llamar en caso de emergencia _____

Haga una lista de todos sus
medicamentos por prescripción
medicamentos sin receta (por ejemplo, aspirina)
vitaminas
hierbas
complementos alimenticios
remedios naturales
cantidad de alcohol que ingiere a diario o a la semana
drogas recreativas

Es importante incluir esta información, en caso de emergencia.
Lleve consigo esta lista. Compártala con su farmacéutico y con las personas que le atienden.

Medicamentos (incluya la cantidad que toma y con cuánta frecuencia y a qué hora del día lo hace)

por prescripción _____

_____

_____

sin receta (por ejemplo, aspirina) _____

_____

_____

This informational brochure can help Spanish-speaking patients better understand how to avoid medication errors. The section "Mi Lista de medicamentos" at one end may be detached and placed in the patient's wallet.

Appropriate Communication for Patients' Age and Development

Children mature at different rates and have different capacities to understand and participate in decisions about their health care. Therefore, not all children of the same age will be able to make the same types of decisions about their care. It is important for caregivers to understand that although living with a chronic or terminal illness can greatly accelerate a child's level of maturity, children who seem capable of making rational decisions still need support from their families. At the opposite end of the age spectrum, elderly patients have their own set of unique considerations.

Infants and Preschool Children

Infants and preschool children cannot make important decisions about their health care. Parents will need to make decisions for them based on what they believe to be in the child's best interests.

Primary School Children

Primary school children may be capable of participating in health care decisions, but a parent should make final decisions about their care. Clinicians should give these children age-appropriate information about their care, with an understanding that children of this age may agree or disagree with their plan of care without fully understanding its implications. Before making any decisions, caregivers should ask for the child's permission and take seriously any strong objections from the child.

Family members who are anxious, stressed, or grieving may need help from the child's providers to focus on what is best for the child. Doing so may be especially difficult when the child has a terminal illness.

Adolescents

Some adolescents have the ability to make the same types of decisions as adults. To ensure that an adolescent is capable of making appropriate health care decisions, caregivers should assess the adolescent's ability to do the following[15]:
- Understand and communicate relevant information
- Think and make choices with a degree of independence
- Assess the potential benefits, risks, and consequences of multiple options

There are unique challenges associated with communicating with adolescents. For example, adolescents may not readily disclose information for fear of being judged. Adolescents are the least likely of all age groups to receive medical care—including prenatal care—and yet are the most likely to engage in high-risk behaviors. Confidentiality is particularly important to adolescents, so they need reassurance that everything they discuss is confidential. When treating adolescents, particularly female patients, it is important that health care professionals provide comfort and show understanding of the patient's needs. All medical procedures should be explained fully before commencing.[15]

The Elderly

Some elderly patients may have cognitive deficits or hearing disabilities, which make communication more challenging. Multiple comorbidities also contribute to miscommunication between caregivers and elderly patients. The following tips from the U.S. National Institute on Aging can help clinicians communicate better with elderly patients[17]:
- Establish respect from the outset by using formal terms of address, such as Mr., Mrs., or Ms.
- Relieve anxiety by asking questions about family or outside interests.
- Introduce yourself clearly.
- Avoid rushing elderly patients. Try to give them enough time to talk about their concerns.
- Beware of any tendencies to minimize complaints, such as "not wanting to be a bother," or concerns about "taking up too much of your time."
- Speak slowly to give patients time to process what is being said.
- Try not to interrupt patients early in the interview. When interrupted, patients are less likely to reveal all their concerns.
- Avoid jargon. Use simple, common language and be willing to ask patients if they understand what you are saying.
- Introduce necessary information by asking patients what they know about their illness and then building on that.
- Assess vision and hearing problems that can affect communication and need to be treated.
- Speak slowly and clearly in a normal tone.
- Face patients directly, at eye level, and keep your hands away from your face while talking, so they can lip-read or pick up visual clues to what you are saying.
- Tell your patients when you are changing the subject. Give clues such as pausing briefly, speaking a little bit more loudly, gesturing toward what will be discussed, gently touching the patient, or asking a question.
- Make sure the setting is adequately lit.
- Ask whether your patients have brought or are wearing the right eyeglasses.

- Make sure your handwritten instructions are easy to read.
- When using printed materials, make sure the type is large enough and the typeface is easy to read.
- Consider using alternatives to printed materials, such as tape-recorded instructions, large pictures or diagrams, or other aids if elderly patients have trouble reading because of either sensory impairment or low literacy skills.

Communicating with Patients with Limited Comprehension and Reading Skills

Appropriate patient education requires effective communication. Many clinicians mistakenly assume that patients can read and understand complex materials.[18] Regardless of a patient's educational or demographic background, it should always be assumed that he or she needs help understanding health conditions and treatment options.

It is also in the organization's best interest to ensure that all patients understand what is being done for them and why. When patients do not understand their treatments, they may become frustrated and uncooperative, which can lead to longer hospital stays, higher health care costs, opportunities for medical errors, and compromised patient safety.

The following tips can be used to help caregivers educate patients with limited reading skills about their care, treatment, and services[19]:

- Use clear communications. All patients should be provided with information that is easy to understand.
- Speak in plain language (*see* Sidebar 4-4 in this chapter and Sidebar 5-9, page 92, in the next chapter).
- Use multiple teaching methods to meet the needs of patients with different learning styles. For example, when educating patients, instead of just providing verbal instructions or giving them written materials, try using pictures, models, audio recordings, or video recordings.
- Fully utilize written materials. Written materials can be made more effective if the provider reads them aloud to the patient while highlighting, underlining, circling, or numbering key points for the patient to remember. Pictograms in written materials can further enhance understanding. For example, a picture of a medication stored in a refrigerator could accompany information about proper storage of insulin (*see* Figure 4-15, page 62). The U.S. Pharmacopeia offers 85 pictograms at http://www.usp.org/audiences/consumers/pictograms.
- For written materials, such as informed consent forms, consult the Readability Toolkit developed by the Group

---

Sidebar 4-4. Key Elements of Plain Language

The key elements of plain language include the following:

- Organize information so that the most important behavioral or action points come first.
- Break complex information into understandable segments.
- Use simple language or define technical terms.
- For written materials, provide ample white space so pages are easier to read.

Source: U.S. Department of Health & Human Services: *Plain Language: A Promising Strategy for Clearly Communicating Health Information and Improving Health Literacy.* Nov. 2005. http://www.health.gov/communication/literacy/plainlanguage/PlainLanguage.htm (accessed Jul. 19, 2010).

Online extras

For links to the Group Health Center for Health Studies Readability Toolkit and the U.S. Pharmacopeia collection of pictograms, visit http://www.jcrinc.com/HCTC10/Extras/.

Health Center for Health Studies in Seattle, Washington (available at http://www.centerforhealthstudies.org/capabilities/readability/ghchs_readability_toolkit.pdf). This toolkit provides substitutions for commonly used words in American English and includes template language that can be adapted for consent forms, thereby lowering the reading level of such written documents.

- Keep patient education information short and specific, and use repetitive messages. Limit patient education to two or three key points. Focus on key behaviors, such as walking for a half hour five times a week or taking the prescribed antibiotic every day for 10 days. Repeat those key points multiple times during the patient visit.

Some organizations also will make follow-up phone calls to patients a few days after teaching to assess learning. The provider might say something like, "I just wanted to make sure everything I told you was clear and to find out how you are doing with the treatments I recommended."[20]

- Take time to assess what the patient has understood. Assessment of learning can be done through the teach-back method or by asking questions that begin with *how* and *what.* For example, the physician might ask about an antibiotic, "How many days in a row do you intend to take

Figure 4-15. U.S. Pharmacopeia Pictogram for Medication Storage

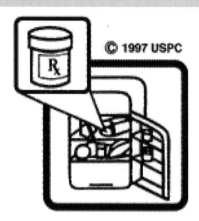

© 1997 USPC

This pictogram can be used in addition to written material and verbal instructions to teach patients about appropriate medication storage. The pictogram shows that the medication should be kept in the refrigerator.

Source: U.S. Pharmacopeia. Used with permission.

your new medication?" to verify that the patient understands that the complete course must be taken. Avoid questions that may elicit only "yes" or "no" responses.

- Spend more time teaching patients who have chronic illnesses. Patients with low health literacy skills often have a difficult time controlling complex chronic illnesses. For example, one study showed that diabetic patients with low health literacy skills had worse glycemic control and higher levels of retinopathy than patients with adequate literacy skills. The same study showed that patients with asthma and low health literacy skills did not know how to use their inhalers properly.[21]

Communicating with Patients with Limited English Proficiency

Organizations in the United States are required by federal law to ensure patient understanding by clearly communicating in ways that are tailored to the individual. Additionally, organizations that receive federal funding are required by the U.S. Centers for Medicare & Medicaid Services (CMS) to comply with civil rights laws prohibiting discrimination against anyone seeking health care services, including those who are blind or deaf or who speak languages other than English.

To comply with CMS requirements, organizations should do the following[22]:

- Assess their populations and language needs.
- Develop a written policy for assessing the needs of individual patients with limited English proficiency.
- Provide free language assistance for those with limited English proficiency.
- Identify effective and convenient resources for language assistance and arrange for these services quickly when needed.
- Hire bilingual staff members who are trained and competent in the skill of interpreting (family or friends of the patient should not be used as interpreters).
- Translate written materials that are routinely given to patients in English.
- Use informed consent forms written in simple sentences in the primary language of the patient.

Patient Education Tool: Understanding Your Doctors and Other Caregivers

As part of its Speak Up campaign (described earlier in Sidebar 4-2, page 55), The Joint Commission has developed an educational tool to help patients who have low health literacy or limited English proficiency. The tool is available in English and Spanish versions (*see* Figures 4-16 and 4-17, pages 64–65 and 66–67, respectively). It includes information about what patients should do if they do not understand what their physician is telling them and what they should do if they cannot read.

Tool for Improving Health Communication

Ask Me 3™ is a tool designed to improve health communication between patients and providers. It was developed by the Partnership for Clear Health Communications at the National Patient Safety Foundation.[23]

The Ask Me 3 initiative provides three simple but essential questions that patients should ask their providers during health care interactions[23]:

1. What is my main problem?
2. What do I need to do?
3. Why is it important for me to do this?

Using the Ask Me 3 approach, providers can do three things to help ensure optimal communication between them and their patients[23]:

1. **Answer 3.** Providers are encouraged not only to educate patients about the Ask Me 3 approach but also to use the

following simple techniques to increase patients' comfort level with asking questions and to help them comply with follow-up instructions after they leave their appointments:

- Create a safe environment where patients feel comfortable talking openly.
- Use plain language instead of technical language or medical jargon.
- Sit down (instead of standing) to achieve eye level with the patient.
- Use visual models to illustrate a procedure or condition.
- Ask patients to "teach back" the care instructions they have been given.

2. **Learn more about low health literacy.** Organizations can use the fact sheets and other communication tools posted on the Ask Me 3 Web site to educate providers about communicating with patients with low health literacy skills.

3. **Incorporate new knowledge into your practice.** Striving to increase knowledge of low health literacy issues and associated concerns can help providers better treat their patients.

An increasing number of organizations are taking an interest in improving health literacy. Many prominent organizations

Online extras

For an Ask Me 3™ poster, visit http://www.jcrinc.com/HCTC10/Extras/.

are partnering with others to develop materials to educate and motivate providers and patients. To educate staff about health literacy issues, organizations can include the Ask Me 3 brochure in patient orientation materials (*see* Figure 4-18, pages 68–69) and can display Ask Me 3 posters in common areas to encourage staff members to discuss the key questions with patients (*see* Online Extras box).

To educate the public about health literacy issues, organizations can do the following[23]:

- Conduct local outreach to promote clear health communication at hospitals and community centers.
- Distribute Ask Me 3 materials and other health literacy information to their constituents.
- Conduct a seminar or panel discussion on health literacy issues at the organization's next convention or meeting.
- Distribute Ask Me 3 brochures at health fairs and events.

Figure 4-16. Understanding Your Doctors and Other Caregivers (English Version)

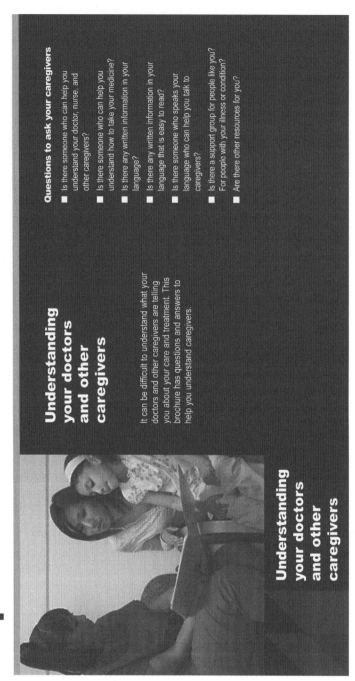

Speak**UP**™

Understanding your doctors and other caregivers

It can be difficult to understand what your doctors and other caregivers are telling you about your care and treatment. This brochure has questions and answers to help you understand caregivers.

Questions to ask your caregivers

- Is there someone who can help you understand your doctor, nurse, and other caregivers?
- Is there someone who can help you understand how to take your medicine?
- Is there any written information in your language?
- Is there any written information in your language that is easy to read?
- Is there someone who speaks your language who can help you talk to caregivers?
- Is there a support group for people like you? For people with your illness or condition?
- Are there other resources for you?

Understanding your doctors and other caregivers

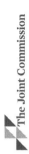

The Joint Commission

(continued on page 65)

Figure 4-16. Understanding Your Doctors and Other Caregivers (English Version), *continued*

What can you do if you don't understand what your caregiver is saying?

Tell them you don't understand. Use body language. If you don't understand shake your head to show that "No, I don't understand." Ask lots of questions. By asking questions you're helping them understand what you need.

What can you do if they explain and you still don't understand?

Tell them you still don't understand. Try to be as clear as possible about what you do not understand. Caregivers have a duty to help you understand. You should not leave until you understand what to do and what is happening to you.

What if the caregiver is rushed and doesn't have time to answer your questions?

Ask them if you need to schedule another appointment when they can answer your questions.

What can you do if you speak another language?

Ask for someone who speaks your language. This person can help you talk to caregivers. This person should work for the hospital or health center. Their job is to help people who speak other languages. This person may not be in the office. He or she may be on the telephone. You have the right to get free help from someone who speaks your language. Ask if there is paper work in your language.

What can you do if you have trouble reading? Or if you cannot read?

Don't be embarrassed. Tell your caregivers. They can help you. They can explain paper work to you. They may even have paper work that is easy to read and understand.

Your doctor's instructions are not clear. Should you try to figure it out yourself?

No. Instructions from your doctor or others are important. Tell them what you think the instructions are. Tell them if they need to write down the instructions. Tell them if you have a family member or friend who helps you take your medicine. Ask the doctor to have someone talk to your family member or friend, too.

What if you don't understand written instructions?

Tell your caregivers. Tell them that you need to have the instructions read to you. Tell them you need instructions that are easy to read. Or that you need instructions in your language.

What can you do if you don't understand the instructions for your medicine?

Tell your doctor if you need help. Tell them what you think the instructions are. Tell them if you don't understand how to take your medicine. Tell them if you don't understand when to take your medicine. Some patients don't understand and take too much or too little of the medicine. That can be dangerous.

How can you remember all of your medicines?

Ask for a card for your medicines. Ask your caregiver to help you write down the medicines and the amount you take. Bring the card with you every time you go to the doctor.

The doctor says I need to have a "procedure." What does that mean?

A procedure can be an operation or a treatment. A procedure can be a test with special equipment. You might be put to sleep or a part of your body might be numbed. Ask questions about what will be done to you. If you speak another language ask for someone who speaks your language. Even if you're in the emergency room you need to understand what will happen to you.

What is informed consent?

Informed consent means that you know how your illness or condition will be treated. It means that you agree to the operation or treatment. It means that you understand the risks. That you know about other treatments available to you. And that you know what can happen if you aren't treated. You will be asked to sign paper work after you agree to the treatment. You need to decide if you will sign or not sign the paper work only after you understand all that was explained to you.

You don't understand the paper work you're given to fill out. What can you do?

Ask caregivers to explain the paper work. Ask them if they can help you fill it out.

Your caregiver asked you to do something that is against your culture or religion. What can you do?

Tell your caregiver about your culture. Or tell them about your religious beliefs. Explain to them what you need to do. When they know what is important to you, they can understand better how to take care of you. There may be a way to meet your caregiver's needs and your needs.

Where can you find more information about your illness or condition?

You can ask another doctor for their opinion. Visit your local library. Ask the people who work at the library for help. If you use a computer, you can look on the Internet. You can try the Medical Library Association by typing in www.mlanet.org/resources/consumr_index.html. Or try Medline Plus by typing in http://medlineplus.gov/. You should talk to your doctor about what you learn.

www.jointcommission.org

The goal of the Speak Up™ program is to help patients become more informed and involved in their health care.

This trifold brochure can help English-speaking patients with low health literacy or limited English proficiency better navigate the health care system.

Figure 4-17. Understanding Your Doctors and Other Caregivers (Spanish Version)

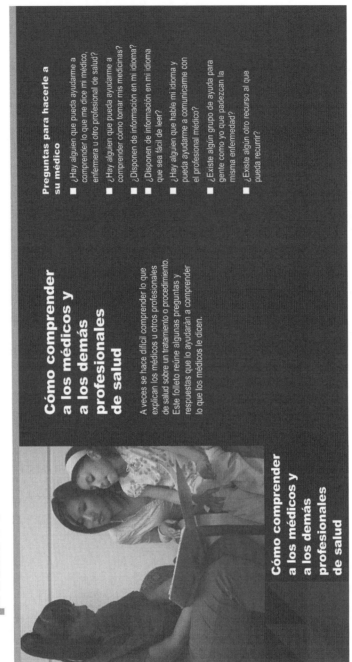

(continued on page 67)

Figure 4-17. Understanding Your Doctors and Other Caregivers (Spanish Version), continued

¿Qué puedo hacer si no comprendo lo que me dicen los profesionales médicos?

Hágales saber que no entiende lo que le dicen. Utilice el lenguaje corporal. Si no entiende algo, diga no con la cabeza para demostrarles que no les entiende. Haga todas las preguntas que necesite. Con sus preguntas les ayudará a entender lo que usted necesita.

¿Qué puedo hacer si con la explicación aún no comprendo?

Dígales que sigue sin comprender. Intente ser lo más claro posible sobre lo que no entiende. Todos los profesionales de salud tienen la obligación de ayudarle a comprender. No se retire del consultorio hasta que no logre comprender lo que le ocurre y lo que debe hacer.

¿Qué ocurre si el profesional de salud está apurado y no tiene tiempo para contestar mis preguntas?

Pregúntele si debe pedir otra cita para que pueda responder a sus preguntas.

¿Qué puedo hacer si hablo otro idioma?

Solicite la presencia de alguien que hable su idioma. Esta persona le ayudará a comunicarse con el profesional. Esta persona debe trabajar para el hospital o centro de salud. Su trabajo es ayudar a las personas que hablan otro idioma. Esta persona podría no estar en la oficina. En este caso, es posible que pueda contactarle por teléfono. Usted tiene derecho a recibir gratuitamente la ayuda de alguien que hable su idioma. Pida que le entreguen folletos en su idioma.

¿Qué puedo hacer si tengo problemas para la lectura o no puedo leer?

No se sienta avergonzado. Informe de su situación a los profesionales médicos. Ellos podrán ayudarle y le leerán lo que dice los folletos. Es posible que cuenten con información que sea fácil de leer y comprender.

Si lo que me indica el médico no me resulta claro. ¿Debo intentar deducir lo que me dice?

No. Las indicaciones del médico son muy importantes. Repita lo que haya comprendido de sus indicaciones. Si lo necesita, pídale que se lo escriba. Infórmele si usted tiene algún familiar o amigo que lo ayuda con las medicinas. Pídale al médico que asigne a alguien para hablar con su familiar o amigo.

¿Qué ocurre si no comprendo las indicaciones escritas?

Informe de su situación a los profesionales médicos. Dígales que necesita que alguien le lea las indicaciones. Dígales que necesita que las indicaciones sean fáciles de leer o que necesita que las indicaciones estén en su idioma.

¿Qué puedo hacer si no comprendo las indicaciones para tomar mis medicinas?

Informe a su médico si necesita ayuda. Repita lo que haya comprendido de sus indicaciones. Hágale saber que no entiende cómo tomar sus medicinas. Hágale saber que usted no entiende cuándo debe tomar sus medicinas. Algunos pacientes no comprenden las indicaciones y toman medicamentos de más o de menos. Esto podría ser muy peligroso.

¿Cómo puedo recordar las medicinas que debo tomar?

Solicite que le entreguen una tarjeta para sus medicinas. Solicítele al médico que le ayude a tomar nota de las medicinas que debe tomar y de la forma en que debe hacerlo. Traiga consigo la tarjeta cada vez que visite a su médico.

El doctor dice que deben hacerme una "intervención". ¿Qué significa esto?

La palabra "intervención" puede usarse tanto para hablar de una operación como de un tratamiento. También puede ser una prueba con un equipo especial. Es posible que lo duerman o que le apliquen anestesia local. Pregunte lo que le van a hacer. Si usted habla otro idioma, solicite la presencia de alguien que hable su idioma. Aunque esté en la sala de emergencias, usted tiene derecho a comprender lo que le harán.

¿Qué es el consentimiento informado?

El consentimiento informado significa que usted sabe cómo se tratará su enfermedad. Significa que usted acepta que se le realice una operación o tratamiento. Significa que usted es consciente de los riesgos, que está al tanto de los tratamientos alternativos y que sabe lo que podría ocurrirle si no se sometiera al tratamiento. Una vez que usted acepte someterse al tratamiento le pedirán que firme unos documentos. Podrá decidir si firmará o no estos documentos sólo después de comprender todo lo que le han explicado.

Si no comprendo la documentación que debo completar. ¿Qué puedo hacer?

Solicite que le expliquen toda la documentación y que le ayuden a completarla.

El médico me ha pedido que haga algo que está en contra de mi cultura o religión. ¿Qué puedo hacer?

Explíquele al profesional acerca de su cultura o de sus creencias religiosas. Explíquele lo que necesita hacer. Sólo cuando logre comprender lo que es importante para usted podrá encontrar la mejor forma de atenderle. Seguramente hay algún modo de hacer coincidir sus necesidades con el tratamiento médico.

¿Dónde puedo encontrar más información sobre mi enfermedad o condición?

Puede solicitar la opinión de otro médico. Acuda a la biblioteca local. Solicite la ayuda de los empleados de la biblioteca. Si tiene computadora, investigue en Internet. Puede visitar el sitio de la Asociación de bibliotecas médicas (Medical Library Association) en www.mlanet.org/resources/consumr_index.html. También puede visitar el sitio de Medline Plus en http://medlineplus.gov/. Comente toda la información nueva con su médico.

www.jointcommission.org

El objetivo del programa "Hable" es ayudar a los pacientes a mantenerse informados y activos durante su atención médica.

This trifold brochure can help Spanish-speaking patients with low health literacy or limited English proficiency better navigate the health care system.

Figure 4-18. Ask Me 3 Brochure

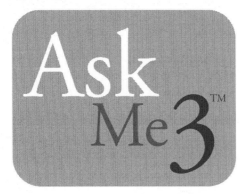

Good Questions for Your Good Health

Every time you talk with a doctor, nurse, or pharmacist,
use the **Ask Me 3** questions to better understand your health.

❶
What is my main problem?

❷
What do I need to do?

❸
**Why is it important
for me to do this?**

When to Ask Questions

You can ask questions when:
- You see your doctor, nurse, or pharmacist.
- You prepare for a medical test or procedure.
- You get your medicine.

What If I Ask and Still Don't Understand?

- Let your doctor, nurse, or pharmacist know if you still don't understand what you need to do.
- You might say, "This is new to me. Will you please explain that to me one more time?"

Who Needs to Ask 3?

Everyone wants help with health information. You are not alone if you find things confusing at times. Asking questions helps you understand how to stay well or to get better.

The **Ask Me 3** questions are designed to help you take better care of your health.
To learn more, visit ***www.npsf.org/askme3***

(continued on page 69)

Figure 4-18. Ask Me 3 Brochure, *continued*

Your Doctor, Nurse, and Pharmacist *Want* to Answer 3

Are you nervous to ask your health provider questions? Don't be. You may be surprised to learn that your medical team wants you to let them know that you need help.

Like all of us, doctors have busy schedules. Yet your doctor wants you to know:

- All you can about your condition.
- Why this is important for your health.
- Steps to take to keep your condition under control.

Asking these questions can help me:

- Take care of my health
- Prepare for medical tests
- Take my medicines the right way

- I don't need to feel rushed or embarrassed if I don't understand something. I can ask my doctor again.
- When I **Ask 3**, I am prepared. I know what to do for my health.

Bring your medicines with you the next time you visit your doctor or pharmacist. Or, write the names of the medicines you take on the lines below.

_____

_____

_____

_____

_____

Like many people, you may see more than one doctor. It is important that your doctors know all the medicines you are taking so that you can stay healthy.

Write Your Doctor's Answers to the 3 Questions Here:

1 What is my main problem?

_____

_____

2 What do I need to do?

_____

_____

3 Why is it important for me to do this?

_____

_____

Ask Me 3™ is an educational program provided by the **Partnership for Clear Health Communication at the National Patient Safety Foundation**™ – a coalition of national organizations that are working together to promote awareness and solutions around the issue of low health literacy and its effect on safe care and health outcomes.

APat2-E 10-07

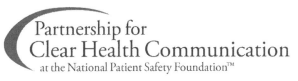

Partnership for
Clear Health Communication
at the National Patient Safety Foundation™

www.npsf.org/askme3

This brochure can help patients become comfortable with asking important questions about their health care.

Source: Partnership for Clear Health Communication at the National Patient Safety Foundation.™ Used with permission.

References

1. Zimmerman P.: Cutting-edge discussions of management, policy, and program issues in emergency care. *J Emerg Nurs* 32:267–268, Jun. 2006.

2. Joint Commission Resources: Q&A: Implementing the SBAR technique. *Perspectives on Patient Safety* 6:8, 12, May 2006.

3. University of Pennsylvania School of Nursing. *Transitional Care Model.* http://www.transitionalcare.info/index.html (accessed Jul. 19, 2010).

4. National Transitions of Care Coalition. *Elements of Excellence in Transitions of Care (TOC): TOC Checklist.* http://www.ntocc.org/Portals/0/TOC_Checklist.pdf (accessed Jul. 19, 2010).

5. Chayboyer W., et al.: *Standard Operating Protocol for Implementing Bedside Handover in Nursing.* Australian Commission on Safety and Quality in Healthcare, 2008. http://www.safetyandquality.gov.au/internet/safety/publishing.nsf/content/com-pubs_CH-BH&WC-con/$File/SOP-Bedside-Handover.pdf (accessed Aug. 22, 2010).

6. Wallis P., et al.: *Standard Operating Protocols for Implementing Whiteboards to Assist with Multidisciplinary Communication on Medical Units.* Australian Commission on Safety and Quality in Healthcare, 2008. http://www.safetyandquality.gov.au/internet/safety/publishing.nsf/content/4C8A959A95F0CD15CA25775400034630/$File/SOP-Whiteboard-Comms.pdf (accessed Aug. 22, 2010).

7. Sidlow R., Katz-Sidlow R.: Using a computerized sign-out system to improve physician–nurse communication. *Jt Comm J Qual Patient Saf* 32:32–36, Jan. 2006.

8. Joint Commission Resources: Focus on five: Strategies to improve hand-off communication: Implementing a process to resolve questions. *Perspectives on Patient Safety* 5:11, Jul. 2005.

9. Van Eaton E., et al.: Organizing the transfer of patient care information: The development of a computerized rounding and sign-out system on continuity of care and resident work. *Surgery* 136:5–13, Jul. 2004.

10. Beresford L.: Change you should believe in. *Hospitalist* 14:1, 14–16, Jul. 2010.

11. Joint Commission Resources: 5 sure-fire methods: Complete and accurate medical records. *The Joint Commission : The Source* 7:2, 5, Apr. 2009.

12. The Joint Commission: *Medication Reconciliation Handbook,* 2nd ed. Oak Brook, IL: Joint Commission Resources, 2009.

13. U.S. Pharmacopeia: Reconciling medications—MEDMARX and meeting a new national patient safety goal. *Medmarx Exchange* Oct. 2004. http://www.usp.org/pdf/EN/patientSafety/mmxExchange2004-10-01.pdf (accessed Feb. 19, 2009).

14. Gebhart F.: Setting up a medication reconciliation system. *Drug Topics,* Jan. 24, 2005. http://drugtopics.modernmedicine.com/drugtopics/article/articleDetail.jsp?id=143478 (accessed Aug. 30, 2010).

15. Joint Commission on Accreditation of Healthcare Organizations: *Patients as Partners: How to Involve Patients and Families in Their Own Care.* Oakbrook Terrace, IL: Joint Commission Resources, 2006.

16. Joint Commission Resources: Strategies for improving health literacy. *The Joint Commission Perspectives on Patient Safety* 8:8–9, Mar. 2008.

17. National Institute on Aging: *Talking with Your Older Patient: A Clinician's Handbook.* National Institute of Health Publication no. 08-7105. Oct. 2008. http://www.nia.nih.gov/HealthInformation/Publications/ClinicianHB (accessed Aug. 22, 2010).

18. Moore C.: Health care literacy and patient safety: The new paradox. In Youngberg B., Hatlie M. (eds.): *The Patient Safety Handbook.* Sudbury, MA: Jones & Bartlett, 2004.

19. U.S. Department of Health & Human Services: *Plain Language: A Promising Strategy for Clearly Communicating Health Information and Improving Health Literacy.* Nov. 2005. http://www.health.gov/communication/literacy/plainlanguage/PlainLanguage.htm (accessed Aug. 22, 2010).

20. Weiss B.: *2007 Health Literacy and Patient Safety: Help Patients Understand,* 2nd ed. Chicago: American Medical Association, 2007.

21. Safeer R., Keenan J.: Health literacy: The gap between physicians and patients. *Am Fam Physician* 72:463–468, Aug. 2005.

22. Wu H., et al.: *Improving Patient Safety Through Informed Consent for Patients with Limited Health Literacy: An Implementation Report.* Washington, DC: National Quality Forum, 2005.

23. Partnership for Clear Health Communication at the National Patient Safety Foundation: *Ask Me 3.* http://www.npsf.org/askme3/ (accessed Jul. 19, 2010).

Chapter 5

Communication in Specific Situations

Chapter 1 discusses issues in communication between providers during transitions of care. This chapter discusses strategies for improving communication between providers during transitions. Sample forms and checklists are provided as available.

Between Primary Care Physicians and Other Specialty Care Providers

When a primary care physician believes that a patient needs care that is outside his or her expertise, he or she may enlist the help of another specialty care provider by requesting either a consultation or a referral (*see* Sidebar 5-1 for essential elements to be communicated prior to consultation or referral). A consultation is a request for an advisory opinion. A referral is a request for the other specialty provider to assume responsibility for managing a patient's condition.[1]

The American Academy of Family Physicians has developed a consultation/referral request form (*see* Figure 5-1, page 72) to help primary care physicians and other specialists communicate better during consultation or referrals. The primary care physician fills out the form and sends it to the subspecialist before the patient's appointment. The form includes instructions about what the primary care physician is asking the subspecialist to do and what type of follow-up information the primary care physician would like to receive from the subspecialist. For example, if the primary care physician is requesting a consultation, he or she may check off or tick the appropriate box on the form asking the subspecialist to confirm diagnosis, to advise as to diagnosis, or to suggest medication or treatment. The primary care physician also may request a follow-up telephone call, periodic status reports, or a written report after the consultation by marking a box on the form.

Between Hospitalists and Other Physicians or Service Units

Patients can be particularly vulnerable during transitions of care between hospitalists and other physicians or service

units. To assist with these transitions of care, hospital medicine programs should develop standardized processes for communication during transitions of care. Key goals for such standardized processes should include the following:
- The process is reproducible.
- The process is interactive (allowing the receiver to review historical information, verify information, and ask questions).
- The information transferred during the process is up-to-date and accurate.

Figure 5-1. Consultation/Referral Request Form

Date:_____

TO: (Consultant's Name)   FROM: (Attending's Name)
         (Address)   (Address)
         (City/State/Zip)   (City/State/Zip)
         (Telephone)   (Telephone)

PATIENT:

_____
     (Name)   (Address)   (Phone)   (Date of Birth)

Tentative Diagnosis:

Requested Disposition:

Consultation *(Please refer patient back for follow-up and treatment.)*   Referral *(Please provide attending physician with summaries of subsequent visits.)*

☐ Confirm diagnosis
☐ Advise as to diagnosis
☐ Suggest medication or treatment

☐ Assume management for this particular problem and return patient after conclusion of care
☐ Assume future management of patient within your field of specialty

If surgery is indicated, attending physician requests to:

☐ Assist   ☐ Give anesthesia
☐ Perform   ☐ Receive status reports of patient's condition

PATIENT INFORMATION
(Pertinent History, Physical and Laboratory Findings, Special Financial Considerations)

Signature:_____

☐ Please call me when you have seen the patient.   Attending Physician
☐ I would like to receive periodic status reports on this patient.
☐ Please send a thorough written report when the consultation is complete.

CONSULTANT'S FINDINGS

☐ I would like to receive periodic status reports on this patient. Signature:_____
                                                   Consultant

Reprinted with permission from the American Academy of Family Physicians, Leawood, Kansas.

This form helps primary care phycisians and other specialists communicate better during consultation or referrals.

Source: American Academy of Family Physicians (AAFP): *Family Medicine in Hospitals,* 5th ed. Leawood, KS: AAFP, 2004. Used with permission.

- The process specifies that the transfer of information take place before, or simultaneous to, the transfer of care responsibility (not afterward).
- The process occurs in an environment that minimizes interruptions (such as background noise, lack of privacy, or interruptions).

Test results are among the key pieces of information to be communicated during transitions of care, particularly if they are critical results. *Critical results* are test results that are abnormal to a degree that it may indicate a life-threatening situation. The Massachusetts Hospital Association and the Massachusetts Coalition for the Prevention of Medical Errors developed a multidisciplinary consensus group of stake-holders in critical results reporting. This group compiled a set of Safe Practice Recommendations that are needed to create a successful critical results reporting system (*see* Sidebar 5-2, page 74).

At Physicians' Transfer of Complete or On-Call Responsibility

As discussed in Chapter 1, poor transitions of care carry substantial risks when physicians are not given adequate information or when they forget or misunderstand information that has been communicated during transitions of care.[2] Many organizations have proposed guidelines for safe and effective transitions of care, which include the following recommendations[3]:

- Receiving physicians should be allotted adequate time for questions.
- It should be clearly conveyed which patients are seriously ill or clinically unstable.
- Transitions of care should include up-to-date information.
- Transitions of care should take place in a quiet atmosphere with minimal distractions.

Verbal interactive communication is the predominant type of communication used during physician transitions of care. During face-to-face transitions, physicians may rely on written, verbal, and nonverbal cues as modes of communi-cation.[4] According to Darrell Solet, M.D., cardiology fellow at the University of Texas Southwestern Medical Center in Dallas, face-to-face communication that is supported by handwritten documentation is the ideal method for physician transitions of care, but he admits that this method may not always be feasible. "The second best method is a phone call," he says. Solet says that when physicians leave written notes or send communications via e-mail, "the receiving physician may miss some important nonverbal aspects to communication. There are subtle messages that you can pick up on by hearing the inflection in someone's voice or watching his or her facial expressions."[5]

The information communicated during physician transitions of care may depend somewhat on the physician's clinical and diagnostic skills. Physicians who have a greater understanding of the patient's clinical conditions and likely contingencies are more likely to focus on relevant information and may be better able to convey that information in a way that promotes a greater understanding by the receiving physician.[4]

Strategies that physicians can use to help foster good communication during transitions of care include the following[2-4]:

- Use face-to-face interaction with time for questions and answers.
- Make sure it is clear to physicians and other care providers when transfer of responsibility takes place.
- Provide a written summary as well as a verbal report.
- Use standardized templates for written reports.
- Provide the incoming physician with recommendations for contingencies if changes to the plan need to be made during an on-call shift.
- Provide a rationale for the plan of care.

Currently, medical residents receive little to no formal training about how to conduct transitions of care; the process is mostly learned informally on the job.[2] However, teaching residents how to conduct transitions of care is critical to quality patient care. Teaching should focus not only on clinical decision making but also on communicating information clearly and efficiently.[4]

Between Anesthesiologists and Postanesthesia Recovery Room Nurses

In the postoperative environment, anesthesiologists and recovery room nurses are involved in multiple transitions of care each day.[6] Because the recovery room tends to be a busy place in which nurses often are involved in multiple tasks at the same time, it is important that nurses set aside time for communication during transitions of care.

When a patient arrives on the postanesthesia care unit (PACU), it is important that the receiving nurse be told how the patient tolerated the procedure and whether the procedure went as planned. The nurse also needs to know whether the patient is hemodynamically stable, whether the patient had any intraoperative complications, what

Sidebar 5-2. Safe Practice Recommendations for Critical Results Reporting

A multidisciplinary consensus group of stakeholders in critical results reporting developed the following questions and answers.

Question: Who should receive critical results?
Answer: The ordering (or responsible) provider and the provider who can take action on the results.

Question: Who should receive the results when the ordering provider is unavailable?
Answer: The organization should create a system that links each patient with a provider or service, a procedure to identify who is responsible when the provider is unavailable, and a central site for call schedules and notification operations.

Question: What results require timely and reliable communication?
Answer: The organization should create a list of values that require notification, including a set with highest priority ("red alert").

Question: When should the results be actively reported to the ordering provider with explicit time frames?
Answer: The organization should have red, orange, and yellow categories of results, each with appropriate notification parameters, and with sequential notification by a prespecified algorithm.

Question: How should the responsible provider be notified?
Answer: The system should involve automatic notification systems for the red category, and the system must ensure receipt by the intended provider.

Question: How can a uniform policy for all types of test results be established?
Answer: The policy development process should involve all the stakeholders, and the culture should provide a sense of teamwork and shared accountability among all the teams involved.

Question: How can reliability be designed into the system?
Answer: The system should force the provider to enter contact information at the time of ordering, and the system should be able to track outstanding tests.

Question: How can the system be supported and maintained?
Answer: The system should include patients and families in test communications, should educate all health care providers about the process, and should monitor the system effectiveness regularly.

Question: How should the infrastructure be supported?
Answer: The hospital should adopt advanced technologies to enhance high-reliability communications and should improve the capabilities of the testing system.

Source: Hanna D., et al.: Communicating critical test results: Safe practice recommendations. *Jt Comm J Qual Patient Saf* 31:62–80, Feb. 2005.

medications were given during the procedure (including time, dose, and therapeutic response), and the patient's current comfort level.[7] Other elements to be included in communication during the transition from the operating room to the postanesthesia care unit include the following[7]:

- Patient name and date of birth
- Procedure performed
- Type of anesthesia administered
- Intravenous fluids administered
- Estimated blood loss
- Surgical site information (dressings, tubes, drains, or packing)
- Airway and oxygenation status
- Thermal status
- Urine output
- Method of pain management

For a sample form for communication during perioperative transitions of care including transfers to the postanesthesia care unit, *see* Figure 5-2, pages 76–77. The form is based on the Situation–Background–Assessment–Recommendation (SBAR) technique discussed in Chapter 4.

Sometimes there is confusion about who is relaying what information to the PACU nurse, which can result in missed or duplicated information. Establishing a standardized approach with specific category prompts can help ensure that important information is being shared and nothing is being overlooked. Clear guidelines should be established regarding what information should be included in each report and who should provide that information.[6] Sidebar 5-3 shows information to include in an anesthesiologist report to the postanesthesia recovery room nurse.

For sample forms for transitions of care from the operating room to the postanesthesia care unit, *see* Figures 5-3 and 5-4, pages 78 and 79, respectively.

Another factor to be considered during transitions of care from the anesthesiologist to the postanesthesia recovery room nurse is the need to limit interruptions as much as possible. Doing so can be challenging in a busy environment, but some organizations have found that many interruptions come from staff rather than from patients. Some examples include someone stopping to say hello, someone asking about the next case, and constant overhead paging. Recognizing where interruptions are coming from is a first step in helping to minimize them.[6]

Sidebar 5-3. Information to Be Included in an Anesthesiologist Report

The following is an example of information that may be included in a report from the anesthesiologist to the postanesthesia recovery room nurse:

- Patient name
- Past medical history
- Past surgical history
- Procedure performed
- Current medications
- Medication allergies
- Anesthesia administered
- Other medications administered
- Anesthesia-related intraoperative course
- Intravenous lines, fluids
- Postanesthesia care unit orders
- Epidural orders

Source: Sullivan E.: Hand-off communication. *J Perianesth Nurs* 22:275–279, Aug. 2007.

At Nursing Shift Changes

Change-of-shift reporting is conducted on every unit in every health care setting several times each day.[8] If communication during a change of shift is ineffective, important information about the patient's plan of care can be overlooked[9] (*see* Sidebar 5-4, page 80, for strategies to improve communication between nurses).

There are several methods for conducting nursing change-of-shift reports, including tape-recorded reports, verbal reports, written reports, or a combination of methods.[10] Some organizations prefer tape-recorded reports because they are streamlined, are cost-effective, and can be replayed if important information is missed during the initial report.[10] However, if tape-recorded reports are used, there must be an opportunity for questions and answers.

Verbal change-of-shift reports are common because they provide an interactive environment and allow for questions and answers. Written reports also can be helpful because they give the receiving nurse documentation of important information.[10] Written and verbal reports often are combined because they allow face-to-face interaction and also provide backup documentation.[10]

Figure 5-2. SBAR Patient Report Guidelines: Perioperative Services

SBAR Patient Report Guidelines: Anesthesia
Provider/OR Nurse to PACU/ICU RN - Worksheet

OR Nurse

S — *Situation*

- ▶ Primary surgeon _____
- ☐ Advance directive, code status _____
- ☐ Infection Control/Isolation _____
- ☐ Family location _____ ☐ Surgical Waiting Room
- ☐ Other:

B — *Background*

- ☐ Primary language spoken
  - ☐ English ☐ Other
- ☐ Belongings disposition ☐ none
  - What: _____
  - ☐ Family _____
  - ☐ Other : _____
- ☐ Communication needs
  - ☐ Hearing Aids ☐ Deaf
  - ☐ Glasses ☐ Blind
- ☐ Communication with family regarding:
  - ▶ Clinical Condition (time) _____
  - ▶ Change in Condition

A — *Assessment*

- ☐ Pre/post skin assessment ☐ WNL
  - Other: _____
- ☐ Preop LOC, neuro assessment
  - ☐ Moves all extremities? _____
  - ☐ AAO x 3? _____
  - ☐ Other: _____
- ☐ Drains
  - ☐ JP, Hemovac X _____ ▶ Location _____
  - ☐ Urology stents, ☐ Rt ☐ Lt ☐ Other _____
  - ☐ Chest tubes ☐ Rt ☐ Lt ▶ cmH2O _____
  - ☐ Penrose, Blake tube X _____ ▶ Location _____
- ☐ Dressings, location, #, any drainage
- ☐ Local used, type, amount, time, location: _____
- ☐ On-Q pump – type local, location: _____
- ☐ Wound Vac orders/settings: _____
- ☐ Medications given on field : See OR record

R — *Recommendation*

- ☐ Post PACU admission _____
- ☐ Specialty bed _____
- ☐ Any Other pertinent _____
- ☐ *Additional Questions/Comments*

Report given to: _____ Time _____

(continued on page 77)

Figure 5-2. SBAR Patient Report Guidelines: Perioperative Services, *continued*

SBAR Patient Report Guidelines: Anesthesia Provider/OR Nurse to PACU/ICU RN - Worksheet

Anesthesia Provider

S *Situation*
- [ ] Patient's name (stamp form)
- [ ] Age _____ Gender M F Height _____ Weight _____
- [ ] Procedure performed: _____

B *Background*
- [ ] Medical History _____
- [ ] Current Diagnosis _____
- [ ] Allergies

A *Assessment*

Current Status - Introp course
- ▶ Type of Anesthesia GA/MAC/Regional _____
- ○ Agents used _____
- ○ Recent narcotics _____
- ○ Antibiotics, time last dose _____
- ○ PONV prevention _____
- ○ Reversal agents given _____
- ○ Vasoactive drips _____
- ○ Other meds given _____
- ▶ IV fluids _____
- ○ Crystalloids _____
- ○ Colloids _____
- ○ Blood products _____
- ▶ IV Access, Lines/Location _____
- ○ Central line (CXR done?) _____   ○ Peripheral IV _____
- ○ Arterial line _____   ○ Swan-Ganz _____
- ○ Cordis _____   ○ CVP _____
- ○ Pacing Wires _____   ○ IABP _____
- ○ Vital Signs _____   ○ Neurologic: LOC _____
- ○ Cardiovascular status, EKG _____
- ▶ Respiratory _____
- ○ O2 _____
- ○ Ventilator settings _____
- ○ Pulse oximetry _____
- ▶ Output _____
- ○ Urine _____
- ○ EBL _____
- ○ NGT

R *Recommendation*
- [ ] Airway plan _____
- [ ] Labs, Xrays to be done _____
- [ ] Pain management plan/issues _____
- [ ] *Additional Questions/Comments (write on reverse)*

Pt Transport ICU - OR

Anesthesia providers will complete the pre-anesthesia assessment and communicate with surgical team any concerns.
The Circulator and the anesthesia provider will go to the ICU when the OR is being prepared.
The Anesthesia Provider will get verbal hand off/report of SBAR form. The Anesthesia provider and surgical team will identify composition of OR transport.
The ICU Nurse, RT, Anesthesia Provider (as required), and Surgical Staff (as required) will transport the patient to the OR red line.
The Anesthesia Provider and Surgical Staff will take the patient beyond the red line to the OR where the Circulator will meet them.

Pt Transport OR-ICU

During the course of the procedure the decision will be made by the Anesthesia Team and the Surgical Team that the patient should be transported directly from the OR to ICU.
Anesthesia Provider will complete the OR to ICU SBAR form and hand it to the Circulator.
Circulator, Anesthesia Provider and Surgical Staff will transport the patient to the ICU.
Anesthesia Provider will provide verbal hand off/report to the ICU Nurse on the elements included on the OR to ICU SBAR form, complete the record and return to the OR.

This form can be used for transitions of care as the patient moves from one perioperative area to the next, including transfers from the operating room to the postanesthesia care unit.

Figure 5-3. SBAR Form for Postanesthesia Care Unit

Situation/Background	Consulting MD's:	Labs & procedures today:	Medication reconciliation
Situation/Background LABEL	Consulting MD's: Other consults: PT / OT / SWS	Labs & procedures today: H/H:_____ BMP:_____ PT:_____ INR:_____	Medication reconciliation Complete / Pending Critical Values:
Diagnosis: History & surgeries:	Diet: Tube feedings:_____ Fluid Restriction & How much:	PTT:_____	**Notes/** **Recommendations:**

Allergies:
 	
VS q:_____
 	
Daily wt:_____
 	
Neuro checks:_____
 	
Foley:_____
 	
I&O:_____
 	
O2: NC / Mask / Treatments:
 	
Accucheck q:_____
	Activity:
	Falls risk: Yes / No
	   Hx falling: Yes / No
	   Morse fall score:_____
	
	Alarms: Yes / No
	
	Sitter: Yes / No
	
	Code status:
	
	Mini Lift:
		Meds & treatments today:
		
		IV fluids:
		
		Blood:
		
		PCA:	

SCD's: Yes / No Drains: Dressings: Discharge planning:	Precautions: Decubitus / Aspiration / Seizure Bleeding / Total Hip / Total Knee Isolation: Type_____	Assessments: Head / Neuro Skin Cardiac Resp GI/GU Ortho IV site / tubing	

NOT PART OF THE MEDICAL RECORD

This form can be used for a patient's transition from the operating room to the postanesthesia care unit.

Source: Doctors Hospital, Baptist Health South Florida, Coral Gables, Florida. Used with permission.

Figure 5-4. Perioperative SBAR Form

S	Patient ID Label Here	Surgeon: Procedure:	Procedure:
		NPO Status: Ht/Wt: Site Marked:	Anesthesia Type: General – Epidural – Spinal – Local – MAC Other:

B			
History: (circle) Other:		Neuro – Seizures - DM – Cardiac Dz – Dysrhythmia – HTN – Resp Dz – Asthma – Renal Dz – Liver Dz – Malignant Hyperthermia	
Allergies:			
Isolation (circle)	MRSA – VRE – TB - Other:		
Cultural/Interpreter:		/ Personal Belongings: Given to:	
Family Contact Info:	Location: Waiting Room – Unavailable Contact #:		

A		ASU →	PSA →	OR → PACU/ASU/CCU
T/HR/BP/RR/SaO2:				
Skin:				
Neuro:				
Pulmonary:				
Cardio/Rhythm/PV:				
GastroIntestinal:				
GU/Cath/Drains:	Circle: Foley – CBI - JPx___ - Hmvac – Other:			
Dressings:				
Musculoskeletal:				
Pain:				
Epidural/Block:				
IV Site & IVF LTC:		Site: LTC:	Site: LTC:	Site: LTC:
Lines (CVL,A-Line):				
Intake/Output & EBL:		I= O=	I= O=	I= O= EBL:
Meds/Reversal Given:				
Infusions:				
Blood Given/Needed:		Given: Needs:	Given: Needs:	Given: Needs:
Abn Labs & Last BS:		BS=	BS=	BS=

R				
BetaBlocker Protocol:		Yes No N/A	Yes No N/A	Yes No N/A
DVT Protocol:		Yes No N/A	Yes No N/A	Yes No N/A
Other:				
Special Equipment:				
Acute Orders:				
Unexpected Events:				
Post Op Destination:		ASU CCU Floor	ASU CCU Floor	ASU CCU Floor
Meds (Antibx) needed		ASU#	CCU	ASU# CCU # Floor Room #

This form can be used as the patient is transferred from one perioperative area to the next, including transfers from the operating room to the postanesthesia care unit.

Source: Parkwest Medical Center. Used with permission.

Nursing reports at the patient's bedside are becoming increasingly common.[10] Advantages to bedside reports include face-to-face interaction, an opportunity for clarification of information, joint interaction with the patient, and visualization of intravenous or incision sites.[10]

The amount of time allocated to the nurses' shift changes is very important. The departing nurses should have enough time toward the end of their shift to fully communicate their information without being in a hurry to leave the organization to go home or do any other personal activity.

The change-of-shift report should include up-to-date information about the patient's health status; the care, treatment, and services provided; and any recent or anticipated changes in the patient's condition. The process should be interactive and provide opportunity for questions and answers.[11]

A standardized approach to transitions of care during nursing shift changes can help ensure that important information is not overlooked (*see* Figure 5-5, page 81, for a checklist of information to be included in nursing change-of-shift reports). Standardized reports can improve the quality and accuracy of information provided. Many organizations now use standardized electronic forms, which allow the patient's critical data to be updated at any time and also provide the nurse who is going off shift with a printout that can serve as the basis for the change-of-shift report.[10] Change-of-shift report tools that are tailored to specific units may also help improve the exchange of information during nursing change of shift (*see* Figure 5-6, page 82, for a sample tool for use by nurses during change of shift).

The SBAR technique can be a helpful tool for nurses to use during change-of-shift reporting. The following example summarizes SBAR[9]:

Situation: The patient's current condition

Background: History of the patient's present illness and any associated history from previous illnesses or hospitalizations

Assessment: Findings from the most recent physical assessment

Recommendations: Recommendations for the patient's continued care, including any outstanding orders that need to be completed

For more information about the SBAR technique, *see* Chapter 4.

Sidebar 5-4. Strategies to Improve Communication Between Nurses

The following strategies can help improve communication between nurses:

- Increase consistency in assigning nurses to the same patients over a number of shifts.
- Structure transitions of care to focus on patient progress rather than on tasks.
- Include physicians in the transition process when feasible.
- Combine the strengths from different styles of communications to develop a communication strategy that meets the needs of the individual patient and the organization or unit.

Source: Boutilier S.: Leaving critical care: Facilitating a smooth transition. *Dimens Crit Care Nurs* 26:137–142, Jul.–Aug. 2007.

Between Nurses and Physicians

As discussed in Chapter 1, nurses and physicians often have distinctly different ways of communicating, so when nurses are communicating with physicians, it is important to remember that the ultimate goal is mutual understanding.[12] When communicating with physicians, nurses should choose their words carefully and be specific about the message they are trying to convey (*see* Sidebar 5-5, page 81, for tips to improve communication from nurses to physicians).

Some important findings that should be included during nurse-to-physician communication include the following:

- The patient's current condition
- Any recent changes in the patient's condition
- Adverse reactions to medications
- Inadequate pain relief
- Abnormal laboratory results
- Any concerns expressed by the patient or family

Before a nurse contacts a physician, the nurse should do the following:

- Visit and assess the patient.
- Discuss the situation with the resource nurse or preceptor, if applicable.
- Review the chart to determine the appropriate physician to call.

Figure 5-5. Handoff Protocol/Checklist

❏ Administrative data
  ❏ Patient name/age/gender/family
  ❏ Date of admission to unit
❏ Problem list
  ❏ Medical history
  ❏ Reason for admission to unit
  ❏ Current medical problems
❏ Current status
  ❏ Neurology: consciousness and sedation score
  ❏ Cardiovascular status: BP, heart rate, and rhythm
❏ Respiratory status: respiratory rate, oxygen saturation, oxygen supplementation, and mechanical ventilation
❏ Medications
  ❏ Regular medications
  ❏ Medications in continuous infusion
  ❏ Feeding
❏ Lines and invasive devices
  ❏ IV lines and fluids input
  ❏ Nasogastric tube and input/output
  ❏ Urinary catheter and urine output
  ❏ Endotracheal tube and secretions

❏ Results
  ❏ Laboratory results
  ❏ Radiology results
❏ Events during the last shift
  ❏ Hemodynamic
  ❏ Respiratory
  ❏ Infection
  ❏ Other
❏ Hands-on checking
  ❏ Running fluids
  ❏ Medications in continuous infusion
  ❏ Mechanical ventilation
  ❏ Monitor alarms
  ❏ Dressings
❏ Tasks expected to be done
  ❏ Laboratory tests and imaging studies (pending results or need to order)
  ❏ Procedures
  ❏ Consultations
  ❏ Others

This checklist can help ensure that important information is not overlooked during a change-of-shift report.

Source: Berkenstadt H., et al.: Improving handoff communications in critical care: Utilizing simulation-based training toward process improvement in managing patient risk. *Chest* 134:158–162, Jul. 2008. Used with permission.

- Know the patient's date of admission and admitting diagnosis.
- Read the most recent progress notes from both the physician and the nurse who worked the previous shift.

Some nurses are intimidated by physicians, but when a nurse has a particular concern about a patient that needs to be passed on to the physician, it is important that the nurse be assertive. Nurses also should not hesitate to ask physicians questions if they do not understand the instructions they have been given regarding the patient's care.[12]

In some cases, it may be helpful for nurses to use written tools, such as the SBAR technique, to aid them in communicating with physicians. For more information about SBAR, *see* Chapter 4.

Sidebar 5-5. Tips for Improving Communication from Nurses to Physicians

To help nurses improve their communication with physicians, nurses can do the following:
- Address the physician by his or her name.
- Have pertinent patient information, including the patient's chart, readily available.
- Clearly express any concern about the patient and the reason for that concern.
- Provide a recommendation or plan for follow-up.
- Focus on the patient problem, not mitigating circumstances.
- Be professional and assertive but not aggressive.
- Continue to monitor the patient problem until it has been resolved.

Figure 5-6. Care Sheet Used During Patient Handover

Affix patient label	Age .... Allergies .... Resuscitation status .... Infection status .... Presenting status .... Presenting problem .... Past medical history .... Diagnosis ....

Admission Date ....

Treatment	Date				
	Time				
Oxygen (%/litres)					
Nebulisers					
Peak flow					
IV/subcutaneous access					
Fluid infusion					
Medication infusion					
Antibiotics (route)					
Fluid balance chart					
Fluid restriction					
Catheter					
Stool chart					
Nasogastric/percutaneous endoscopic gastrostomy regimen					
Vomiting					
Special diet					
Food chart					
Observations: irregularities and interventions					
Last blood glucose (mmol)					
Pain score (1-3, high = pain)					
Wounds					
Pressure areas intact					
Mobility status					
Mouth care					
Referrals to other practitioners					
Estimated transfer/discharge date					
Estimated transfer/discharge location					
Planned/investigations					
Remarks					
Signature					

This tool helps nurses exchange information during change of shift.

Source: Davies S., Priestley M.: A reflective evaluation of patient handover practices. *Nurs Stand* 20:49–52, Feb. 2006. Used with permission.

For their part, physicians should regard nurses as valued members of a health care team whose common goal is the best possible care for the patient. Often nurses have spent more time with the patient than the physician has, and thus nurses may be the first to notice changes in the patient's condition that could signal a problem. Physicians should understand that inquiries from nurses stem from concerns about the patient and are not intended as challenges to the physicians' authority or expertise. Physicians should calmly and respectfully listen to nurses' concerns and be willing to help address the situation.

There are times when disruptive clinician behavior can interfere with effective communication between nurses and physicians. Disruptive behavior, which the American Medical Association defines as "personal conduct, whether verbal or physical, that negatively affects or potentially may affect patient care including, but not limited to, conduct that interferes with one's ability to work with other members of the healthcare team," can have a negative impact on quality care and patient safety.[13] Because disruptive behavior has recently been recognized as a growing concern that needs to be addressed,[13] Joint Commission standards now require that organizations have a code of conduct that specifically defines acceptable and disruptive and inappropriate behaviors. The standards also require that leaders create and implement a process for managing disruptive and inappropriate behaviors. The Joint Commission also has issued a *Sentinel Event Alert* on behaviors that undermine a culture of safety (*see* Sidebar 5-6).

Changes in long-standing patterns of ineffective communication between nurses and physicians will not occur without the support of organization leadership. Leaders must seek to provide education for both nurses and physicians that will help them discard those old, unproductive patterns and find new ways to work more cooperatively. A number of organizations have developed successful strategies for making positive changes in the relationship between nurses and physicians, including the following[14]:

- Zero-tolerance policy regarding disrespectful or disruptive behavior
- Clearly enforced code of conduct
- Process for promptly addressing complaints
- Establishment of a nurse-physician liaison group that meets regularly to discuss problems
- Program in which medical students follow and observe nurses as part of their training, thereby gaining a better understanding of nurses' role

---

Sidebar 5-6. Joint Commission *Sentinel Event Alert* on Behaviors That Undermine a Culture of Safety

In July 2008, The Joint Commission issued a *Sentinel Event Alert* on behaviors that undermine a culture of safety. Intimidating and disruptive behaviors described in the alert include both overt actions, such as verbal outbursts and physical threats, and passive activities, such as refusing to perform assigned tasks or quietly exhibiting uncooperative attitudes during routine activities. According to the alert, health care professionals in positions of power often manifest such intimidating and disruptive behaviors as reluctance or refusal to answer questions or impatience with questions, reluctance or refusal to return phone calls or respond to pages, and use of condescending language or voice intonation. Root causes and contributing factors of intimidating and disruptive behaviors are examined in the alert, and The Joint Commission recommends 11 specific actions for organizations to take to address such behaviors in an effort to create and maintain a culture of safety.

The full text of the *Sentinel Event Alert* is available at http://www.jointcommission.org/SentinelEvents/ SentinelEventAlert/sea_40.htm.

- Special code to signal additional staff members to help contain the situation when unacceptable behavior occurs
- Web-based program for collecting reports of disruptive behavior, including those submitted anonymously, and passing them through appropriate channels for action to be taken

Between the Emergency Department and Another Department or Unit Within the Hospital

Effective communication during transitions of care between the emergency department (ED) and other units can help reduce the amount of time unit nurses and receiving physicians spend looking for information at a later stage in the patient's care[15] (*see* Sidebar 5-7, page 84, for a list of key information that may be exchanged during the transition from the emergency department to the inpatient unit).

Sidebar 5-7. Key Information to Exchange During a Transition from the Emergency Department to Another Unit

The following information can help with continuity of care during a patient transition from the emergency department to an inpatient unit:

- Patient name/identification number
- Patient's date of birth
- Reason for emergency department visit
- Relevant past medical history
- Medications/allergies
- Results of diagnostic and laboratory tests (or note to check back if pending)
- Emergency department chart
- Emergency contact information
- List of patient's property

Source: McFetridge B., et al.: An exploration of the handover process of critically ill patients between nursing staff from the emergency department and the intensive care unit. *Nurs Crit Care* 12:261–269, Nov.–Dec. 2007.

If inpatient units are not getting the information needed when patients are transferred from the emergency department, constructive feedback should be provided to the ED staff. This feedback should specify what information is necessary but not being received, along with related errors or adverse outcomes.[16]

Another strategy that might help improve communication between the emergency department and inpatient units is to improve the electronic availability of important information such as current vital signs, physician orders, progress notes, pending test results, and which physician is currently responsible for the patient. Organizations also should have mechanisms in place for assigning patient responsibility, particularly for patients who are "boarding" (being kept in the emergency department until a bed becomes available), and expectations for each specialty should be clearly defined.[16]

Between Two Separate Specialty Care Facilities

Hospital and Long Term Care

As noted in Chapter 1, transitions of care between hospital emergency departments and long term care facilities can be challenging because the resident has caregivers in five different domains during one episode of emergency care[17]:

1. The nursing home before the emergency department visit

2. The ambulance on the way to the emergency department
3. The emergency department
4. The ambulance on the way back from the emergency department
5. The nursing home after the emergency department visit

There also are multiple processes taking place during the transition through each domain. For example, the following exchange processes occur when transitioning a patient from a long term care facility to the hospital emergency department[18]:

- The long term care facility contacts Emergency Medical Services (EMS) to transport the patient from the facility to the hospital.
- EMS picks up the patient and begins recording patient information, including any care provided or observations during transport.
- EMS notifies the hospital that the patient is being transported.
- EMS brings the patient to the hospital.
- Key personnel are assigned to the patient (for example, physician, nurse, case manager, social worker).
- Patient information is collected and transferred to a physician order form.
- The physician confirms the orders and signs them.
- Medications are reconciled.
- Patient care is provided, and then the patient is transferred to an inpatient unit or back to the long term care facility.

The following exchange processes occur when transitioning a patient from a hospital to a long term care facility[18]:

- The hospital notifies the long term care facility that the patient is being transported.
- The hospital contacts Emergency Medical Services to transport the patient from the facility to the hospital.
- EMS picks up the patient and begins recording patient information, including any care provided or observations during transport.
- EMS brings the patient to the long term care facility.
- The nurse at the long term care facility receives and assesses the patient.
- The physician orders and discharge summary are transcribed into the physician order form.
- The record is reviewed for omissions.
- The physician is called to approve the orders.

To improve transitions between the long term care facility and the hospital, each person involved in a patient exchange should know his or her role in the process. Expectations should be established for the health care team sending the patient and for the team receiving the patient.[19] The National Transitions of Care Coalition (NTOCC) has developed a proposed framework for measuring transitions of care (*see* Figure 5-7, page 86) that can help organizations define roles and processes.

Many hospitals and long term care facilities have developed and implemented standardized forms and processes to help improve communication during transitions of care. An advantage to standardized forms is that the long term care facility, the Emergency Medical Service staff, and the emergency department staff all receive a familiar, concise form that can be easily completed during transitions of care. Such a form eliminates the need to search through pages of documents to locate essential information.[17]

Emergency department physicians and nurses have reported that the use of standardized forms made it easier to understand the patient's presenting problem, compile the patient's medication list, and expedite the gathering of information.[17] Figure 5-8, page 87, shows a form for transfer of a patient from a nursing home to a hospital. Figure 5-9, page 88, shows a resident information checklist for receiving patients from a hospital to a long term care facility.

Michael LaMantia, M.D., and colleagues conducted a literature search to find out what types of interventions have successfully improved communication during transitions of care between nursing homes and hospitals.[20] The following five studies were reviewed[20]:

1. In South Australia, a study was conducted to determine whether a medication transfer summary, combined with an assisted medication review after discharge, would help improve appropriate medication use. At patient discharge, the medication transfer summary was sent to the nursing home. The summary was followed by a conference between the hospital and the receiving organization to review medications within 14 days after patient discharge. At the end of the study, it was determined that appropriateness of medication use was improved.

2. A U.S. hospital in New York conducted a study to determine whether pharmacist-performed medication reconciliation would decrease medication errors after discharge. Following the study, only 2.3% of patients experienced an adverse drug event related to a medication discrepancy, compared to 14.5% before the pharmacist-performed medication reconciliation was initiated.

3. A U.S. study in North Carolina was conducted to evaluate the use of a one-page transfer document for transferring nursing home patients to the hospital emergency department. The document included information about the patient's medication regimen. At the end of the study, 88% of the emergency department providers surveyed said that the list of medications had made caring for the patient "a lot easier."

4. A U.S. end-of-life care study conducted in Oregon was intended to evaluate the effectiveness of a physician order form for life-sustaining treatment. The study followed 180 nursing home residents who did not want to be resuscitated, or who wanted to be transferred to the hospital only if comfort measures failed. At the end of the 12-month study, only 13% of participants had been hospitalized. None had been resuscitated.

5. A U.S. study conducted in Indiana attempted to determine whether a one-page emergency department transfer form could help improve information being provided during transfer from a nursing home to the hospital emergency department. Following the study, successful documentation (defined as 9 of 11 pieces of medical information) increased from 58.5% to 77.8%.

Hospital and Home Care

It is sometimes difficult for hospital-based providers to anticipate the needs of home care providers during transitions of care if they have never worked in the home health care environment.[21] The National Transitions of Care Coalition encourages the use of case managers to coordinate care during the transition from hospital to home. According to the NTOCC, case managers can assist patients during transitions of care by acting as patient advocates, assessing adherence to medication regiments and treatments, helping motivate patients, and coordinating necessary outside care resources. Case managers also can assist caregivers during transitions of care by making sure that the appropriate people have access to the patient's medication list and advanced directives. Case managers can provide caregivers with information about the patient's ability and willingness to adhere to medication and treatment regimens, health literacy status, understanding of self-care, and functional or cognitive limitations.[19]

For organizations that do not use a case management approach to transitions between the hospital and home care, hospital-based caregivers may need guidance from home health caregivers regarding what information needs to be shared. Such information may include the following[21]:

- Diagnosis
- Reason for referral to home care

Figure 5-7. NTOCC Proposed Framework for Measuring Transitions of Care

I. <u>Structure</u>

    A. **Accountable provider at all points of transition.** Patients should have an accountable provider or a team of providers during all points of transition. This provider(s) should be clearly identified and will provide patient-centered care and serve as central coordinator of his/her care across all settings, across other providers.

    B. **Plan of Care.** The patient should have an up-to-date, proactive care plan that includes clearly defined goals, takes into consideration the patient's preferences, and is culturally appropriate.

    C. **Use of health information technology (HIT).** Management and coordination of transitional care activities is facilitated through the use of integrated electronic information systems that are interoperable and available to patients and providers.

II. <u>Processes</u>

    A. **Care Team processes**
- Medication reconciliation
- Test tracking (lab and diagnostic procedures)
- Referral tracking
- Admission and discharge planning
- Follow up appointment

    B. **Information transfer/communication between providers**
- Timeliness, completeness, and accuracy of information transferred
- Protocol of shared accountability in effective transfer of information

    C. **Patient education and engagement**
- Patient prepares for transfer
- Patient education for self-management
- Appropriate communication with patients with limited English proficiency and health literacy

III. <u>Outcomes</u>
- Patient experience (including family or caregiver)
- Provider experience (individual practitioner or health care facility)
- Patient safety (medication errors, etc.)
- Health care utilization and costs (reduced avoidable hospitalization)
- Health outcomes (clinical and functional status, intermediate outcomes, therapeutic endpoints)

This framework can help both long term care facilities and hospitals include all pertinent information when transferring patients from one facility to the other.

Source: National Transitions of Care Coalition (NTOCC): *Improving on Transitions of Care: How to Implement and Evaluate a Plan.* Little Rock, AR: NTOCC, 2008. Used with permission.

Figure 5-8. Nursing Home–to–Hospital Transfer Form

Patient transfer to hospital from:_____

Name of Nursing Home

To: ☐ Coliseum ☐ MCCG ☐ Northside ☐ Other Date: _____	
Name: Sex: ☐ F ☐ M	
D.O.B.	
Attending physician: **Code Status:**	
Copy of advance directives included: ☐ Yes ☐ No	
Last vitals (date& time): Temp: _____ P _____ R _____ BP _____ / _____	
Allergies/sensitivities:	
Chief complaint/reason for transfer:	
Mental status: ☐ Oriented time/place ☐ Confused ☐ Dementia ☐ Cooperative ☐ Uncooperative ☐ Alert ☐ Wanders ☐ Unable to communicate ☐ Requires soft restraints	
Diet: ☐ Feeds self ☐ Requires assistance	
Activity: ☐ Ambulates without assistance ☐ Ambulates with some assistance ☐ Bedrest ☐ Uses assistive devices ☐ Cane ☐ Walker ☐ Other:	
History of falling ☐ Yes Date: ☐ No **Prosthetics:** ☐ Dentures ☐ Glasses ☐ Artificial Limbs	
Date of last BM:	

Current Medication	Dose	Frequency	Route	Last Dose

*Include vitamins/supplements etc.

Vaccines: Flu ☐ Yes Date: ☐ No   **Pneumonia** ☐ Yes Date: ☐ No   **Tetanus** ☐ Yes Date: ☐ No
Personal effects:
Skin breakdown: ☐ Yes   ☐ No   Location:
Other health information that will assist with care of patient:
Nearest relative: Contacted by phone: ☐ Yes   ☐ No
Name of person completing form: **Contact number:**
Reprinted with permission from Medical Center of Central Georgia, Macon, Georgia.

This form can be used for a transition of care from nursing home to hospital.

Source: Medical Center of Central Georgia, Macon, Georgia. Used with permission.

Figure 5-9. Resident Information Checklist from ED/Hospital

Resident Name

Date and time of transfer

❑ Resident discharge summary

❑ List of pending test results

❑ List of pending appointments

❑ Medication list, including time of last dose, stop dates for new medications

❑ List of all treatments received by resident during hospital stay

❑ Consultant notes

❑ Vital signs during hospital stay

❑ Hospital contact name and phone or pager number

The following information is documented in the medical record:

❑ Verbal communication between NF and hospital within 24 hours

Contact name: _____ time:_____

❑ Verbal communication regarding the resident's return to the NF provider

❑ Evidence of medication reconciliation with prehospitalization MAR

❑ Verbal communication with family/LAR within 24 hours of return to the facility.

Contact name: _____ time:_____

Name completing form

Date

This checklist can help nursing facility (NF) staff members ensure that they have received the information they need to continue the patient's care.

Source: National Transitions of Care Coalition (NTOCC): *Improving on Transitions of Care: How to Implement and Evaluate a Plan.* Little Rock, AR: NTOCC, 2008.

- A list of providers who will be responsible for the patient's care following hospital discharge and contact information for each provider
- An assessment of the patient's functional and cognitive status
- A reconciled postdischarge medication list
- Information about how the patient will obtain medications and treatment supplies following discharge
- Dietary or activity restrictions
- Teaching done prior to discharge
- Emergency contact information
- Follow-up appointment dates and times

Between Specialty Care Provider or Primary Care Physician and Pharmacy

With the number of medications on the market today, there are many potential opportunities for breakdowns in communication between prescribers and pharmacists. Incomplete medication orders, medications with look-alike/sound-alike names, and orders with illegible handwriting all can contribute to miscommunication between prescribers and pharmacists.

To reduce communication errors related to look-alike/sound-alike medications, both prescribers and pharmacists should develop policies for giving and receiving verbal orders. An example of a policy for verbal orders might be that when a prescriber issues a verbal order, he or she states the order and dosage slowly and clearly and then spells the name of the medication. The pharmacist then repeats the order back to the physician, again spelling the name of the medication.

Illegible handwriting also contributes to errors related to look-alike/sound-alike medications. To reduce errors related to illegible handwriting, physicians should consider writing orders slowly and carefully, printing in neat block letters, rather than hastily scrawling in script or cursive.[22]

Prescribers should use only standardized acronyms, abbreviations, and symbols for prescription orders. The Joint Commission has developed a list of abbreviations that should not be used (*see* Figure 5-10, page 90). Joint Commission International (JCI) requires that organizations have a standardized list of specific abbreviations that should not be used, but the organization determines which particular abbreviations appear on its list.

In organizations such as hospitals, where prescribers and pharmacists are all part of the same health care system,

computerized prescriber order entry (CPOE) systems can help reduce errors due to poor verbal or written communication. However, such systems must be used properly and consistently or they can introduce new errors.

Used correctly, CPOE helps prevent transcription errors, and most systems are also equipped with decision support tools for prescribers. For example, CPOE systems can alert prescribers to potential medication allergies, drug interactions, duplicate orders, dosages prescribed that are smaller or larger than what is considered normal, and other unusual situations.

When CPOE is not an option, physicians and pharmacists should have systems in place to ensure that all orders received are complete. According to the National Coordinating Council for Medication Error Reporting and Prevention, complete prescription orders should include the following[23]:
- Name of medication (both brand name and generic)
- Exact metric weight or concentration
- Dosage form
- Age and, when appropriate, weight of the patient
- Clear, specific directions for use
- A brief notation of purpose (for example, "for cough"), unless considered inappropriate for purposes of maintaining confidentiality

At Discharge from Hospital

Discharge planning should begin well in advance of the patient's discharge, possibly even as early as admission. Discharge planning includes educating the patient and family about the patient's diagnoses, medications, and follow-up orders. In addition, the patient should be assessed for decision-making ability and the ability to comprehend discharge instructions.[24]

When preparing a patient for discharge, the nurse, in collaboration with the case manager and social worker, should ascertain whether the patient has physical barriers to continuing care, such as lack of transportation to follow-up appointments or lack of appropriate equipment or supplies at home.[24] If the patient needs assistance with transportation or equipment, referrals should be made to community-based agencies that provide the necessary resources or services. Home health care should also be arranged, if warranted.[25]

If a patient is being transferred to another facility, the nurse should contact the receiving facility to discuss the patient's

Figure 5-10. The Joint Commission Official "Do Not Use" List

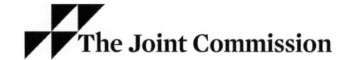
The Joint Commission

Official "Do Not Use" List[1]

Do Not Use	Potential Problem	Use Instead
U (unit)	Mistaken for "0" (zero), the number "4" (four) or "cc"	Write "unit"
IU (International Unit)	Mistaken for IV (intravenous) or the number 10 (ten)	Write "International Unit"
Q.D., QD, q.d., qd (daily)	Mistaken for each other	Write "daily"
Q.O.D., QOD, q.o.d, qod (every other day)	Period after the Q mistaken for "I" and the "O" mistaken for "I"	Write "every other day"
Trailing zero (X.0 mg)* Lack of leading zero (.X mg)	Decimal point is missed	Write X mg Write 0.X mg
MS	Can mean morphine sulfate or magnesium sulfate	Write "morphine sulfate" Write "magnesium sulfate"
MSO$_4$ and MgSO$_4$	Confused for one another	

[1] Applies to all orders and all medication-related documentation that is handwritten (including free-text computer entry) or on pre-printed forms.

*Exception: A "trailing zero" may be used only where required to demonstrate the level of precision of the value being reported, such as for laboratory results, imaging studies that report size of lesions, or catheter/tube sizes. It may not be used in medication orders or other medication-related documentation.

The abbreviations on The Joint Commission's official "Do Not Use" list above should not be used for prescribing.

plan of care and any follow-up measures that will be necessary to meet the patient's ongoing needs. A written discharge summary and current medication list should also be sent to the receiving facility.

Prior to discharge, the nurse and the patient should discuss the following[25]:
- The patient's current condition
- Any potential symptoms, problems, or changes that may occur after release from care and what to do if these do occur
- Medications that the patient will be taking and any potential interactions or side effects. The patient should be given a written medication list with specific instructions about how to take each medication and information about possible side effects. The nurse should then ask the patient to demonstrate how to take the medications.
- Signs and symptoms of infection
- Whom to call if questions or problems arise

One tool that is being used to incorporate such discussion and thereby improve the quality of the hospital discharge process is called Project RED (*see* Sidebar 5-8, page 91). The letters *RED* stand for *Re-Engineered Discharge*. For further details about the development of Project RED, including illustrations of key elements, *see* the case study in Chapter 7.

Another major effort to improve the hospital discharge process is called Project BOOST (Better Outcomes for Older adults through Safe Transitions). The Project BOOST case study in Chapter 7 provides a detailed description of the development and implementation of this program. In 2008, the year Project BOOST began, six sites participated. Twenty-four more sites joined the program in 2009. By mid-2010, an additional 36 sites had joined.[26] The program continues to expand, including the launch of a BOOST community site to facilitate communication among participating hospitals and, beginning in fall 2010, a tuition-based model of the program.[26]

When patients are discharged from the hospital, they often lack the knowledge and resources to adequately participate in their own care. According to the National Transitions of Care Coalition, improving patient education will create better-informed consumers, which in turn will improve transitions of care.[19]

One strategy that specialty care providers can use to improve patient education is to speak in plain language (*see* Sidebar 5-9, page 92; *see also* Sidebar 4-4 in Chapter 4, page 61). Providers should avoid the use of specialized medical terminology when possible, or they should define the medical terms using simple words and short sentences.[27]

To help patients better understand discharge instructions, specialty care providers should have a variety of teaching methods ready to meet the needs of patients with different learning styles. These methods include verbal instructions, written materials, video recordings, models, pictures, audio recordings, and drawings.[28]

Some organizations have developed tools or checklists to help coordinate transitions of care between specialty care providers and patients and families (*see* Figure 5-11, pages 93–95). Key points to be included in transition-of-care tools include the following[19,21]:

- Diagnosis
- Treatment options
- Follow-up care
- Medications, including potential side effects or complications
- Who is responsible for which aspects of the patient's care
- What information will be shared with other providers and within what time frame
- What resources are available to assist the patient after discharge

Sidebar 5-8. Project RED

The Project RED (Re-Engineered Discharge) intervention is a patient-centered, standardized approach to discharge planning and discharge education, initially developed through research funded by the Agency for Healthcare Research and Quality (AHRQ), the lead federal agency charged with improving the quality, safety, effectiveness, and efficiency of health care. AHRQ recently has funded Joint Commission Resources (JCR) to provide customized training and technical assistance to several health systems implementing the Project RED intervention in their hospitals. Project RED aims to improve the patient's preparedness for self-care and to reduce the likelihood of readmission.

The Project RED intervention redesigns the work-flow process and improves patient safety by using a discharge advocate who follows 11 discrete, mutually reinforcing action steps shown to improve the discharge process and decrease hospital readmissions. The three key elements of the Project RED intervention include the discharge advocate, the after-hospital care plan, and a follow-up phone call to the patient by a clinical pharmacist a few days after discharge, intended to review medications.

Patients who have a clear understanding of their after-hospital care instructions, including how to take their medicines and when to make follow-up appointments, are 30% less likely to be readmitted or to visit the emergency department than are patients who lack this information.

Whenever possible, patients should be involved in their care, including their discharge planning (*see* Sidebar 5-10, page 96, for opportunities for patient and family involvement).

Patient Continuity of Care Questionnaire

The Patient Continuity of Care Questionnaire (*see* Figure 5-12, pages 97–99) is a tool developed in Canada by members of the Department of Psychology at the University of Regina in Regina, Saskatchewan, and members of the Department of Medicine at Lakeshore General Hospital in Pointe-Claire, Quebec. It contains questions about the information patients received before hospital discharge as well as questions about

Sidebar 5-9. Plain Language

Plain language uses simple words and phrases. Consider the following changes to simplify the way you write and speak English with patients.

Instead of	Try
assist	help
discontinue	stop
indication	sign
in the event of	if
maximum	greatest, largest, most
minimum	least, smallest
modify	change
notify	tell
necessitate	cause, need
objective	goal
optimum	best, greatest, most
perform	do
provide	give, offer, say
purchase	buy
regarding	about, of, on
remain	stay
request	ask
require, requirement	need
retain	keep
submit	give, send
subsequent	next
subsequently	later
sufficient	enough
transmit	send
utilize	use
validate	confirm
with reference to	about

Source: PlainLanguage.gov: *Simple Words and Phrases.* http://www.plainlanguage.gov/howto/wordsuggestions/ simplewords.cfm (accessed Aug. 25, 2010).

follow-up after discharge. The questionnaire was mailed to orthopedic inpatients who had multiple care providers and family medicine inpatients with multiple comorbidities 4 weeks after hospital discharge. At the same time, charts were reviewed for information about length of stay, home care after discharge, educational materials provided, and readmissions.[29]

Findings from analysis of the questionnaire showed several areas for improvement of continuity of care. For example, 50% of the patients surveyed reported that they had not been properly informed about resources, educational materials, and other forms of support available to help them maintain continuity of care. And 30% said that at discharge they were not given key information, such as whom to contact if they experienced nonurgent symptoms after discharge.[29]

Patient Education Tool: Planning Your Follow-Up Care

As part of its ongoing Speak Up™ campaign (*see* Sidebar 4-3 in Chapter 4, page 55), The Joint Commission developed a two-page educational brochure, available in English and Spanish, to help patients prepare for discharge (*see* Figures 5-13 and 5-14, pages 100–101 and 102–103, respectively). It includes questions that patients should ask about their condition and their medications. (Another educational brochure from the Speak Up campaign, "Help Avoid Mistakes with Your Medicines," which includes a wallet-size medication list the patient can carry, appears in English and Spanish versions as Figures 4-13 and 4-14 in Chapter 4.)

Within Specific Types of Nonhospital Settings
Behavioral Health Care

Several types of transitions of care occur in behavioral health care facilities, including change-of-shift report, transfer of care from one team to another, transfer of care from one provider to another, transfer between units, and transfer between facilities. Some behavioral health facilities use more than one communication method during transitions of care, such as verbal reports, written reports, recorded reports, patient notes, and standardized forms.[30]

In an ideal situation, transitions of care would be done face-to-face in a quiet environment with minimal interruptions. Realistically, other methods of communication may be necessary to ensure that the appropriate information is transferred in a timely manner. When face-to-face communication is not possible, there should be a method in place that will allow for questions and answers. Key personnel should be involved in determining what information should be shared during transitions of care. Such information includes the following[30,31]:

- Diagnoses
- Medical and psychiatric history
- Current vital signs
- Pending results of diagnostic or laboratory tests
- Current medications
- Results of most recent mental status exam

Figure 5-11. Personal Health Record Booklet

Personal Health Record

This is the Personal Health Record of

If you have questions or concerns,

Contact _____

at (____) _____ - _____

**REMEMBER
to take this Record with you
to all your doctor visits**

Personal Information

Address:

Home Phone #:
Alternate Phone #:
Birth Date:
Advance Directive/Living Will: __ Yes __ No
Where located?

Caregiver Information
Name:
Relation to Patient:
Home Phone #:
Alternate Phone #:

Provider Information

Primary Care Doctor:
Phone #:
Pharmacy:
Other Providers:

_____

_____

_____

_____

Questions for my Primary Care Doctor:

(continued on page 94)

Figure 5-11. Personal Health Record Booklet, *continued*

Personal Goal	**Medical History and Red Flags**

Notes for my Primary Care Doctor:

Recent Hospitalization:

Reason for Hospitalization:

Discharge Checklist

Before I leave the care facility, the following tasks should be completed:

❑ I have been involved in decisions about what will take place after I leave the facility.

❑ I understand where I am going after I leave this facility and what will happen to me once I arrive.

❑ I have the name and phone number of a person I should contact if a problem arise during my transfer.

❑ I understand what my medications are, how to obtain them and how to take them.

❑ I understand the potential side effects of my medications and whom I should call if I experience them.

❑ I understand what symptoms I need to watch out for and whom to call should I notice them.

❑ I understand how to keep my health problems from becoming worse.

❑ My doctor or nurse has answered my most important questions prior to leaving the facility.

❑ My family or someone close to me knows that I am coming home and what I will need once I leave the facility.

❑ If I am going directly home, I have scheduled a follow-up appointment with my doctor, and I have transportation to this appointment.

This tool was developed by Dr. Eric Coleman, UCHSC, HCPR, with funding from the John A. Hartford Foundation and the Robert Wood Johnson Foundation

(continued on page 95)

Figure 5-11. Personal Health Record Booklet, *continued*

To better manage my health and medications, I will...

- Take this Personal Health Record, with me to wherever I go, including ALL doctor visits and future hospitalizations.

- Call my doctor if I have questions about my medications or if I want to change how I take my medications.

- Tell my doctors about ALL medications I am taking, including over-the-counter drugs, vitamins and herbal formulas.

- Update my Medication Record with any changes to my medications.

- Know why I am taking each of my medications.

- Know how much, when and for how long I am to take each medication.

- Know possible medication side effects to watch out for and what to do if I notice any.

Medication Record

Medication & Supplement Record

Name	Dose	Reason	New?

Allergies:

Notes and Questions for My Primary Care Doctor:

This booklet can provide caregivers with the patient's medical history and medications.

Source: This Personal Health Record is a key component of the Care Transitions Intervention™ developed by the Care Transitions Program (http://www.caretransitions.org) with the generous support of the John A. Hartford Foundation. Used with permission.

Sidebar 5-10. Opportunities for Patient and Family Involvement in Patient Care and Discharge Planning

- Provide information to patients about their medical conditions and treatment care plan in a way that is understandable to them.
- Make patients aware of their prescribed medications, dosages, and required time between medications.
- Inform patients who the responsible provider of care is during each shift and whom to contact if they have a concern about the safety or quality of care.
- Provide patients with the opportunity to read their own medical record as a patient safety strategy.
- Create opportunities for patients and family members to address any medical care questions or concerns with their health care providers.
- Inform patients and family members of the next steps in their care, so they can if necessary communicate this information to the care provider on the next shift, or so they are prepared to be transferred from one setting to the next or to their home.
- Involve patients and family members in decisions about their care at the level of involvement that they choose.

Change-of-shift reports may also include overnight admissions and any problems encountered during the previous shift.[30]

Long Term Care

Good communication between nurses and physicians in long term care facilities can have a profound effect on the quality of a resident's care.[32] Therefore, interventions to improve communication within long term care facilities must target both nurses and physicians.[33] As with most health care organizations, staff members in the long term care setting have busy schedules, so it is important for organization leaders to find ways to improve communication without increasing staff work load.[32]

In one study, one important recommendation made by nurses to foster good communication is for physicians to treat nurses with respect. A respectful attitude includes a willingness on the part of the physician to admit that the nurse may know more about some residents than the physician does; therefore, it is important that physicians listen to what nurses have to say without interrupting.[33]

When calling a physician about a resident, nurses should be prepared. Nurses should organize the information they want to convey and should research any diagnoses, conditions, or medications with which they are unfamiliar.[34]

When nurses contact physicians to discuss a resident's care, it is important that the nurses communicate clearly by explaining their reason for calling and by clearly stating what

they want from the physician.[33] The use of standardized tools, such as SBAR, can help nurses communicate resident-related information in a concise manner.[34]

Nurses in long term care facilities often find it difficult to reach physicians when clinical issues need to be addressed. To increase the likelihood of reaching the physician when calling about a resident's care, long term care nurses should consider doing the following[34]:
- Identifying key personnel in the physician's office and developing a collegial relationship
- Asking contacts in the physician's office the best time and method for reaching the physician
- Giving office managers enough information for the physician to make a clinical decision when he or she is not available to speak on the phone
- Asking for the physician's cell/mobile phone or pager number

Because both nurses and physicians have busy schedules, nurses should try to reduce the number of phone calls they make to physicians. Strategies to reduce the number of calls include bundling calls to prevent redundancy, addressing resident issues while the physician is in the facility, and postponing calls until the next business day, when appropriate.[33]

Interventions to Reduce Acute Care Transfers (INTERACT II) is a quality improvement program for nursing homes that is supported by a grant from the Commonwealth Fund, a private foundation that aims to promote a high-performing health care system that achieves better access, improved quality, and greater efficiency. The purpose of the

Figure 5-12. Patient Continuity of Care Questionnaire

Study ID #: _____

Patient Continuity of Care Questionnaire (PCCQ)

INSTRUCTIONS: These statements are designed to assess the care you received around the time of discharge from hospital. Please complete on your own or with assistance. An informal caregiver (e.g., family, friends) can also complete on behalf of a patient.

Read each statement and circle a number between 1 and 5 to indicate whether you 1 (strongly disagree), 2 (somewhat disagree), 3 (cannot decide whether you agree or disagree), 4 (somewhat agree), or 5 (strongly agree) with the statement.

How strongly do you agree or disagree with this statement?	Strongly Disagree	Somewhat Disagree	Hard to Decide	Somewhat Agree	Strongly Agree	Not Applicable
BEFORE DISCHARGE						
1. I was provided with clear information on my diagnosis.	1	2	3	4	5	NA
2. I was provided with clear information on my prognosis.	1	2	3	4	5	NA
3. I was told about non urgent symptoms that may occur and how I should cope with these	1	2	3	4	5	NA
4. I was given information on symptoms that may signal a need to seek urgent medical attention & whom to contact for these symptoms (e.g. specialist, family physician, homecare).	1	2	3	4	5	NA
5. I was told about clinical findings that may impact my future health or care (e.g. history of blood clots, cancer, high blood pressure).	1	2	3	4	5	NA
6. I was given complete information on my medications (e.g., type, purpose, how given, when, how often for hour long, how much, side effects, drug interactions, nature and frequency of blood work).	1	2	3	4	5	NA
7. I was given dietary instructions (e.g., requirements, restrictions, instructions to plan daily meals).	1	2	3	4	5	NA
8. I was provided with information on recommendations and restrictions in activities, exercises and aids.	1	2	3	4	5	NA
9. I was given information on medical equipment and supplies (e.g., what needed, whom to contact).	1	2	3	4	5	NA
10. I was given information on follow-up appointments that have been made for me and appointments I have to schedule for myself.	1	2	3	4	5	NA
11. I was given written information on recommended support services (e.g., Home Care, Respite, Adult Day Program) and target date for initial contact.	1	2	3	4	5	NA

(continued on page 98)

Figure 5-12. Patient Continuity of Care Questionnaire, *continued*

Study ID #: _____

How strongly do you agree or disagree with this statement?	Strongly Disagree	Somewhat Disagree	Hard to Decide	Somewhat Agree	Strongly Agree	Not Applicable
12. I was informed of ongoing treatment that may be required after discharge (e.g., purpose, how, when) and whether I will have ongoing contact with providers of my care (e.g., physician, etc.).	1	2	3	4	5	NA
13. I was informed of patient resources/supports (e.g., peer support groups) that may be available.	1	2	3	4	5	NA
14. I was informed of different self management tools and educational material (e.g., diaries, books, tapes, videos) that could be helpful to me.	1	2	3	4	5	NA
15. My informal caregivers (e.g., family, friends) were given information on resources/support (e.g., peer support groups, community organizations).	1	2	3	4	5	NA
16. My informal caregivers had the necessary information about my health that they needed in order to help me out.	1	2	3	4	5	NA
17. Providers understood my expectations, beliefs and preferences.	1	2	3	4	5	NA
18. I felt "known" (e.g. current clinical condition and events) by the providers involved in my care.	1	2	3	4	5	NA
19. I had confidence in the providers involved in my care.	1	2	3	4	5	NA
20. I was satisfied with the information from the providers involved in my care.	1	2	3	4	5	NA
21. I was satisfied with the emotional support from the providers involved in my care.	1	2	3	4	5	NA
22. I was satisfied with the opportunity to talk and raise questions with the providers involved in my care.	1	2	3	4	5	NA
23. The different providers appeared to communicate well with each other while I was in hospital/convalescent care.	1	2	3	4	5	NA
24. A well-developed and realistic follow-up plan was prepared and explained to me.	1	2	3	4	5	NA
25. I was involved in and agreed with the follow-up plan.	1	2	3	4	5	NA
26. My family was involved in follow-up as appropriate.	1	2	3	4	5	NA
27. I felt adequately prepared for discharge.	1	2	3	4	5	NA

(continued on page 99)

Figure 5-12. Patient Continuity of Care Questionnaire, *continued*

Study ID #: _____

How strongly do you agree or disagree with this statement?	Strongly Disagree	Somewhat Disagree	Hard to Decide	Somewhat Agree	Strongly Agree	Not Applicable
AFTER DISCHARGE						
28. I feel "known" (e.g. current health condition) by my present providers who have taken over my care since discharge.	1	2	3	4	5	NA
29. I have confidence in my present providers who have taken over my care since discharge.	1	2	3	4	5	NA
30. I am satisfied with the information from my providers who have taken over my care since discharge.	1	2	3	4	5	NA
31. I am satisfied with the emotional support from my providers who have taken over my care since discharge.	1	2	3	4	5	NA
32. I am satisfied with the opportunity to talk and raise questions with my providers who have taken over my care since discharge.	1	2	3	4	5	NA
33. As far as I am aware, the different health care providers in hospital have communicated well with those in the community about my care.	1	2	3	4	5	NA
34. As far as I am aware, my family physician or other key provider was contacted and informed about the important aspects of care that I received (e.g. diagnosis, prognosis, treatment, medications, etc.).	1	2	3	4	5	NA
35. I have reviewed my overall treatment plan with my family physician since my discharge.	1	2	3	4	5	NA
36. The follow-up plan has been followed or adjusted as necessary.	1	2	3	4	5	NA
37. I was given consistent information by all providers about my care.	1	2	3	4	5	NA
38. I was reminded about important appointments (e.g., letter, phone call).	1	2	3	4	5	NA
39. As far as I am aware, necessary forms were all completed.	1	2	3	4	5	NA
40. As far as I am aware, necessary forms were sent to all appropriate places/providers.	1	2	3	4	5	NA
41. As far as I am aware, no forms or information were lost when I was discharged.	1	2	3	4	5	NA

This questionnaire can help organizations target areas for improvement during the transition from hospital to home.

Source: Oxford University Press in association with the International Society for Quality in Health Care. Used with permission.

Figure 5-13. Planning Your Follow-Up Care (English Version)

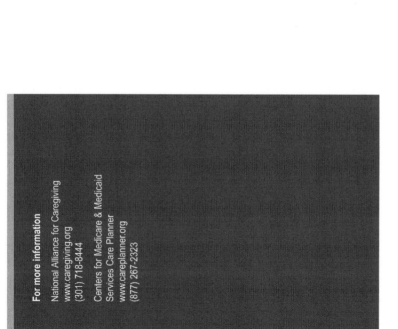

(continued on page 101)

Figure 5-13. Planning Your Follow-Up Care (English Version), *continued*

Before leaving the hospital, you should be given written instructions about your follow-up care. This brochure provides questions to help you get the information you need for the best follow-up care.

What should you do before leaving the hospital?

☐ Find out if the hospital has a discharge planner, social worker or nurse who can help you plan your follow-up care.

☐ Ask a family member or friend to help plan your follow-up care.

☐ Take a notepad to the hospital that you can write questions, answers and reminders on.

What if you have trouble understanding the language used in the instructions?

Ask for a translation or an interpreter.

You feel overwhelmed by the follow-up care you need. What can you do?

Ask about referrals for home care services or a skilled nursing facility. Find out about payment options, including whether financial assistance is available. Find out if the service or organization is licensed or accredited. Organizations accredited by The Joint Commission are listed on Quality Check at www.qualitycheck.org.

Questions to ask about your condition

☐ How soon should you feel better after leaving the hospital?

☐ Will you be able to walk, climb stairs, go to the bathroom, prepare meals and drive?

☐ Are there any special instructions for daily activities? For example, should you take a shower instead of a bath?

☐ How much help will you need after you leave the hospital? Should someone be with you 24 hours a day?

☐ What signs and symptoms should you watch for? If you have them, what should you do?

☐ Will you need any special equipment at home? Where can you get the equipment? Is it covered by your insurance, Medicare, or other health plan?

☐ Will you need physical therapy? Are there any physical exercises you need to do? If so, get written instructions.

☐ If you have wounds, how do you take care of them? How long should it take them to heal?

☐ Will you need to have any follow-up tests? Who should you follow up with to get the test results?

☐ Will you need to schedule any follow-up visits with your doctor?

☐ When can you expect to go back to work?

☐ Who can you call if you have any problems after leaving the hospital?

Questions to ask about your medicines

☐ What medicines will you need to take at home? Get a written list that includes all of your medicines—new and old. Take this list with you when you go for follow-up care.

☐ Can you get written instructions about your medicines? Make sure you understand the instructions. Ask any questions before you leave the hospital.

☐ Are there any medicines, vitamins or herbs that you should not take with your medicines?

☐ Are there any foods and drinks—including alcohol—that you should avoid while you're taking your medicines?

☐ Are there any side effects of your medicines? What should you do if you have side effects?

www.jointcommission.org

The goal of the Speak Up™ program is to help patients become more informed and involved in their health care.

This trifold brochure can help English-speaking patients be involved in their discharge planning.

Figure 5-14. Planning Your Follow-Up Care (Spanish Version)

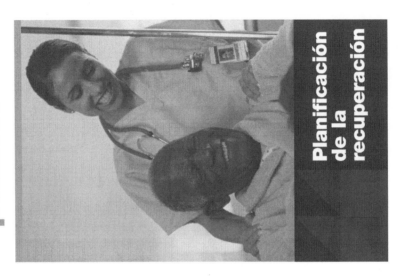

¡Hable!

Planificación de la recuperación

Si desea obtener información más detallada, visite:

National Alliance for Caregiving
www.caregiving.org
(301) 718-8444

Centers for Medicare & Medicaid
Services Care Planner
www.careplanner.org
(877) 267-2323

The Joint Commission

(continued on page 103)

Figure 5-14. Planning Your Follow-Up Care (Spanish Version), *continued*

Antes del alta, se le darán instrucciones por escrito acerca de la atención durante la recuperación. Este folleto contiene la información que necesita para lograr el mejor cuidado mientras se recupera.

¿Qué debo hacer antes del alta?
□ Averigüe si el hospital cuenta con un planificador de alta, trabajador social o personal de enfermería que le pueda ayudar con la planificación de su recuperación.
□ Pídale a un familiar o amigo que le ayude a planificar su recuperación.
□ Lleve una libreta al hospital para que pueda escribir las preguntas, respuestas y recordatorios.

¿Qué puedo hacer si tengo dificultades para entender el idioma usado en las instrucciones? Pida una traducción o la ayuda de un intérprete.

Me siento agobiado por el proceso de recuperación que necesito realizar. ¿Qué puedo hacer?
Pida referencias para servicios de atención médica en casa o una organización de servicios de enfermería especializados. Averigüe acerca de las opciones de pago, y si existe la posibilidad de ayuda financiera. Infórmese si el servicio u organización cuenta con una licencia o acreditación. Las organizaciones que cuentan con la acreditación de el Joint Commission se enumeran en Quality Check en www.qualitycheck.org.

Preguntas que debe hacer acerca de su condición
□ ¿Qué tan pronto me sentiré bien después del alta?
□ ¿Podré caminar, subir escaleras, ir al baño, preparar comida y conducir?
□ ¿Qué instrucciones especiales hay sobre las actividades cotidianas? Por ejemplo, ¿debo tomar una ducha en vez de un baño en tina?
□ ¿Que tipo de ayuda necesitaré cuando me den el alta? ¿Necesitaré atención las 24 horas del día?
□ ¿A cuáles síntomas debo prestar mayor atención? En caso de tener alguno, ¿qué hago?
□ ¿Necesitaré algún equipo especial en casa? ¿Dónde puedo conseguir este equipo? ¿Está cubierto por mi seguro, Medicare u otro seguro médico?
□ ¿Tendré que hacer terapia de rehabilitación física? ¿Necesitaré realizar algún ejercicio físico? En caso de que sea así, pida que le den instrucciones por escrito.
□ En caso de que tenga alguna herida, ¿qué procedimiento debo seguir para tratarla? ¿En cuánto tiempo sanará?
□ ¿Tendré que realizarme algún examen de seguimiento? ¿Con quién debo ponerme en contacto para obtener los resultados de estos exámenes?
□ ¿Debo programar una consulta de seguimiento con el médico?
□ ¿Cuándo podré regresar al trabajo?

□ ¿A quién puedo llamar si tengo algún problema después del alta?

Preguntas que debe hacer acerca de sus medicinas
□ ¿Qué medicamentos tendré que tomar en casa? Haga una lista por escrito que incluya todas sus medicinas, ya sean nuevas o viejas. Llévela consigo cuando tenga alguna cita relacionada con su proceso de recuperación.
□ ¿Puedo obtener instrucciones por escrito acerca de mis medicinas? Asegúrese de entender las instrucciones. Haga todas las preguntas que necesite antes del alta.
□ ¿Existe alguna vitamina, medicamento o hierba que debo evitar mientras tome mis medicinas?
□ ¿Debo evitar alguna comida o bebida (incluyendo alcohol) cuando tome mis medicinas?
□ ¿Las medicinas tienen algún efecto secundario? ¿Qué hago si sufro alguno de éstos?

www.jointcommission.org

El objetivo del programa "Hable" es ayudar a los pacientes a mantenerse informados y activos durante su atención médica.

This trifold brochure can help Spanish-speaking patients be involved in their discharge planning.

Sidebar 5-11. INTERACT II Tools

Communication Tools
- Early Warning Tool ("Stop and Watch")
- Early Warning Tool, Spanish ("Pare Y Observe")
- Early Warning Tool, Creole ("Pran Tan Gade")
- Instructions for Early Warning Tool
- SBAR Communication Tool and Progress Note (*see* Figure 5-15, pages 105–106)
- Instructions for SBAR Communication Tool and Progress Note
- Change in Condition File Cards
- Instructions for Change in Condition File Cards and Care Paths
- Resident Transfer Form (*see* Figure 5-16, pages 107–108)
- Acute Care Transfer Envelope with Checklist (*see* Figure 5-17, page 109)
- Instructions for Resident Transfer Form and Acute Care Transfer Envelope with Checklist (*see* Figure 5-18, pages 110–111)

Care Paths
- Dehydration

- Fever
- Mental Status Change
- Symptoms of CHF [congestive heart failure]
- Symptoms of Lower Respiratory Infection
- Symptoms of UTI [urinary tract infection]
- Instructions for Care Paths and Change in Condition File Cards

Advance Care Planning Tools
- Overview of Advance Care Planning Tools
- Advance Care Planning Communication Guide
  - Part 1: Tips for Starting the Conversation
  - Part 2: Communication Tips
  - Part 3: Helpful Language for Discussing End of Life Care
- Residents at High Risk of Entering Actively Dying Process
- Examples of Comfort Care Interventions
- Understanding Advance Directives
- "What Is Palliative Care?" Brochure
- Artificial Nutrition and Hydration at End of Life
- Instructions for Advance Care Planning Tools

Source: INTERACT II: *Working Together to Improve Care and Reduce Acute Care Transfers (Home Page)*. 2010. http://interact.geriu.org/ (accessed Aug. 22, 2010).

INTERACT II program is to reduce the frequency of resident hospital admissions. At the program's core is a set of tools designed to do the following[35]:
- Help staff members quickly identify a change in a resident's status
- Ensure that staff members conduct a comprehensive assessment when a change in resident status is noted
- Improve documentation related to a change in resident status
- Improve communication between providers

The INTERACT II tools are grouped into three categories[35]: (1) communication tools, (2) care paths or clinical tools, and (3) advance care planning tools. (*See* Sidebar 5-11 for a complete list of INTERACT II tools. The INTERACT II tools shown in Figures 5-15 through 5-18, pages 105–111, can also be accessed online at http://interact.geriu.org/.)

Home Care
Support from home care services can help patients with recovery after hospitalization and decrease readmissions.

Communication within home care facilities is not limited to communication among home care providers. It also includes contact with the facility that is transferring the patient and with the patient's primary care physician. Home care agencies should discuss in advance what information they require during a transition of care with representatives from local hospitals and work with them to develop standardized methods of communication. Part of that communication should include clear instructions about which physician is responsible for the patient's care after discharge.[36] Home care agencies also may want to consider adding a pharmacist to their team to identify and resolve patient-related medication issues and to assist with medication reconciliation.[37]

When patients are readmitted to the hospital, home care agencies should share information about the patient's home care, including the patient's medication list, with the hospital.[36]

The Home Health Quality Improvement Campaign is a U.S. Centers for Medicare & Medicaid Services initiative to

Figure 5-15. SBAR Communication Tool and Progress Note

SBAR
Physician/NP/PA Communication and Progress Note

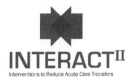

INTERACT^{II}
Interventions to Reduce Acute Care Transfers

Before Calling MD/NP/PA:
- ☐ **Evaluate the resident**, complete the SBAR form (use "N/A" for not applicable)
- ☐ **Check VS:** BP, pulse, respiratory rate, temperature, pulse ox, and/or finger stick glucose if indicated
- ☐ **Review chart** (most recent progress notes and nurse's notes from previous shift, any recent labs)
- ☐ **Review an *INTERACT II Care Path or Acute Change in Status* File Card** if indicated
- ☐ **Have relevant information available when reporting** (i.e. resident chart, vital signs, advanced directives such as DNR and other care limiting orders, allergies, medication list)

S SITUATION

This is_____(nurse) I am calling about_____(Resident's name)
The problem/symptom I am calling about is _____
The problem/symptom started_____
The problem/symptom has gotten (circle one) worse/better/stayed the same since it started
Things that make the problem/symptom worse are _____
Things that make the problem/symptom better are_____
Other things that have occurred with this problem/symptom are_____

B BACKGROUND

Primary diagnosis and/or reason resident is at the nursing home _____
Pertinent medical history/include recent falls, fever, decreased intake/fluids, CP, SOB, other

Mental Status or Neuro changes: (Y/ N: confusion/agitation/lethargy) Temp _____ BP _____
Pulse rate/rhythm _____ Resp rate _____ Lung Sounds_____
Pulse Oximetry_____ % On RA _____ on O2 at _____ L/min via _____ (NC, mask)
GI/GU changes (nausea/vomiting/diarrhea/impaction/distension/decreased urinary output)_____
Pain level/location/status_____
Change in function/intake/hydration _____
Change in Skin Color_____ Wound Status (if applicable)_____
Labs _____
Medication changes or new orders in the last two weeks _____
Advance Directives (Full code, DNR, DNI, DNH, other, not documented)_____
Allergies_____ Any other data_____

A ASSESSMENT (RN) or APPEARANCE (LPN)

(For RNs): What do you think is going on with the resident? (e.g. cardiac, infection, respiratory, urinary, dehydration, mental status change?) I think that the problem may be _____ - *OR*
I am not sure of what the problem is, but there had been an acute change in condition.
(For LPNs): The patient appears _____ (e.g. SOB, in pain, more confused)

R REQUEST

I suggest or request:
- ☐ Provider visit (MD/NP/PA)
- ☐ Monitor vital signs (Frequency_____) and observe
- ☐ Lab work, xrays, EKG, other tests _____
- ☐ Medication changes _____
- ☐ New orders _____
- ☐ IV or SC fluids_____

Staff name_____ **RN/LPN**
Reported to: Name _____ **(MD/NP/PA) Date_ /_/_____ Time_____** am/pm
If to MD/NP/PA, communicated by: ☐ Phone   ☐ Fax (attach confirmation)   ☐ In person
Patient name _____

(Please see Progress Note on back of this Form)

(continued on page 106)

Figure 5-15. SBAR Communication Tool and Progress Note, *continued*

Progress Note

Signature:_____RN / LPN   Date:____/____/_____   Time:____:_____ AM / PM

Return call/new orders from MD/NP/PA: Date:____/____/_____   Time:____:_____ AM / PM

This tool can assist with communication between nurses and physicians regarding a change in a resident's status.

Source: © 2010 Florida Atlantic University. The INTERACT II Tools, educational materials, and implementation strategies were developed by Drs. Joseph Ouslander, Gerri Lamb, Alice Bonner, and Ruth Tappen, and Laurie Herndon, and colleagues in a project supported by the Commonwealth Fund based at Florida Atlantic University. Initial versions of the INTERACT Tools were developed by Dr. Ouslander and colleagues at the Georgia Medical Care Foundation with the support of a special study contract from the Center for Medicare & Medicaid Services. Used with permission.

Figure 5-16. Resident Transfer Form

RESIDENT TRANSFER FORM
INTERACT^II

SENT TO: *(Name of Hospital)*
_____

SENT FROM: *(Name of Nursing Home)*
_____

Date:___/___/_____ Unit: _____

RESIDENT:
Last Name   First Name   MI

DOB:___/___/___
Language: ☐English ☐Other:_____
Resident is: ☐SNF/rehab ☐Long-term

CONTACT PERSON:
(Relative, guardian or DPOA/Relationship)
_____ name

Is this the health care proxy?   ☐Yes ☐No
Telephone:(   )_____ - _____
Notified of transfer: ☐Yes ☐No
Aware of diagnosis: ☐Yes ☐No

CODE STATUS:
☐DNR ☐DNH ☐DNI ☐Full Code

MD/NP/PA IN NURSING HOME:
☐MD ☐NP ☐PA
_____ name
Telephone:( )__-_____ Pager:( )__-____

WHO TO CALL TO GET QUESTIONS ANSWERED ABOUT THE RESIDENT?
_____ name _____ title Telephone:( )___ - _____

REASON FOR TRANSFER *(i.e., What Happened?)*

List of Diagnoses:_____

VS: BP___ HR___ RR___ T___ pOx___ FS glucose ___ Time Taken:___:___ AM/PM
Allergies:_____ Tetanus Booster *(date)*:___/___/_____
Usual Mental Status:
☐ Alert, oriented, follows instructions
☐ Alert, disoriented, but can follow simple instructions
☐ Alert, disoriented, but cannot follow simple instructions
☐ Not alert

Usual Functional Status:
☐ Ambulates independently
☐ Ambulates with assistance
☐ Ambulates with assistive device
☐ Not ambulatory

Please see SBAR form for additional information

DEVICES / SPECIAL TREATMENTS:
☐ IV/PICC line
☐ Pacemaker
☐ Foley Catheter
☐ Internal Defibrillator
☐ TPN
☐ Other:_____

AT RISK ALERTS:
☐ None   ☐ Seizure
☐ Falls   ☐ Harm to:
☐ Pressure   ☐ Self ☐ Others
  Ulcer   ☐ Restraints
☐ Aspiration ☐ Limited/non-weight
☐ Wanderer   bearing: ☐Left ☐Right
☐ Elopement ☐ Other:

ISOLATION / PRECAUTION:
☐MRSA   ☐VRE
☐C-Diff
☐Other:_____
Site:_____
Comment:_____

CAPABILITIES OF THE NURSING HOME TO CARE FOR THIS RESIDENT:
☐ IVF therapy   ☐IV antibiotics   ☐MD/NP/PA follow up visit within 24 hours
☐ Q shift monitoring by an RN   ☐ Other:_____

NURSING HOME WOULD BE ABLE TO ACCEPT RESIDENT BACK UNDER THE FOLLOWING CONDITIONS:
☐ ED determines diagnosis, and treatment can be done in NH   ☐ VS stabilized and follow up
☐ Other: _____   plan can be done in NH

Form Completed By:
_____ name _____ title _____ signature
Report Called In By: Report Called To:
_____ name _____ title _____ name _____ title

(continued on page 108)

Figure 5-16. Resident Transfer Form, *continued*

RESIDENT TRANSFER FORM
ADDITIONAL INFORMATION
(may be faxed to ED/hospital within 7-12 hours)

INTERACT^{II}
Interventions to Reduce Acute Care Transfers

RESIDENT NAME:

Last: _____ First: _____ MI: ___ DOB: ___/___/___

Date Transferred to the Hospital: ___/___/___

TREATMENTS AND FREQUENCY:	SKIN / WOUND CARE:
(*include special treatments such as dialysis, chemo-therapy, transfusions, radiation, TPN, hospice*)	High risk for pressure ulcer: ☐ Yes ☐ No Pressure ulcers: (*stage, location, appearance, treatments*) Wound care sheet attached: ☐ Yes ☐ No

IMMUNIZATIONS:	DIET:
Influenza Date: ___/___/___	Needs assistance with feeding: ☐ Yes ☐ No Trouble swallowing: ☐ Yes ☐ No
Pneumococcal Date: ___/___/___	Special consistency: (*thickened liquids, crush meds, etc.*)
Tetanus Tet-Diphtheria Date: ___/___/___	Tube feeding: ☐ Yes ☐ No

PHYSICAL THERAPY	ADLs:
Resident is receiving therapy with goal of returning home: ☐ Yes ☐ No - or - Patient is LTC placement: ☐ Yes ☐ No Weight bearing status: ☐ Non-weight ☐ Partial weight ☐ Full weight Fall risk: ☐ Yes ☐ No Interventions: _____	(*mark I=independent; D=dependent; A=needs assistance*) _____ Bathing _____ Dressing _____ Toileting/Transfers _____ Ambulation _____ Eating _____ Can ambulate _____(distance) with _____(assistive device or I)

DISABILITIES:	IMPAIRMENTS:	CONTINENCE:
(*amputation, paralysis, contractures*)	(*cognitive, speech, hearing, vision, sensation*)	☐ Bowel ☐ Bladder Last bowel movement: Date: ___/___/___

BEHAVIORAL or SOCIAL ISSUES and INTERVENTIONS:

FAMILY ISSUES:	PAIN ASSESSMENT:

SOCIAL WORKER:	REASON FOR ORIGINAL SNF ADMISSION:
_____ name Telephone:( ) _____ - _____	Bed hold: ☐ Yes ☐ No

This form can assist with communication between the nursing home and the hospital.

Source: © 2010 Florida Atlantic University. The INTERACT II Tools, educational materials, and implementation strategies were developed by Drs. Joseph Ouslander, Gerri Lamb, Alice Bonner, and Ruth Tappen, and Laurie Herndon, and colleagues in a project supported by the Commonwealth Fund based at Florida Atlantic University. Initial versions of the INTERACT Tools were developed by Dr. Ouslander and colleagues at the Georgia Medical Care Foundation with the support of a special study contract from the Center for Medicare & Medicaid Services. Used with permission.

Figure 5-17. Acute Care Transfer Envelope with Checklist

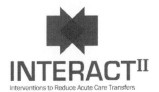

INTERACT^{II}

Interventions to Reduce Acute Care Transfers

ACUTE CARE TRANSFER DOCUMENT CHECKLIST

RESIDENT NAME _____

COPIES SENT WITH RESIDENT (Check all that apply):

These documents should ALWAYS accompany patient:

_____ Resident Transfer Form

_____ Face Sheet

_____ Current Medication List or Current MAR

_____ Advance Directives

_____ Care limiting Orders

_____ Out of hospital DNR

_____ Bed hold policy

Send these documents IF INDICATED:

_____ SBAR/Nurse's Progress Note

_____ Most Recent History & Physical and any recent hospital discharge summary

_____ Recent MD/NP/PA Orders related to Acute Condition

_____ Relevant Lab Results

_____ Relevant X-Rays

_____ PERSONAL BELONGINGS SENT WITH RESIDENT:

     _____ Eyeglasses _____ Hearing Aid _____ Dental Appliance

     _____ Other (specify)

Signature of ambulance staff accepting envelope: _____

(Please make a copy and keep this for your records in the nursing home)

This checklist can help nursing home workers ensure that all relevant documents accompany the resident when he or she is transferred from the nursing home to the hospital.

Source: © 2010 Florida Atlantic University. The INTERACT II Tools, educational materials, and implementation strategies were developed by Drs. Joseph Ouslander, Gerri Lamb, Alice Bonner, and Ruth Tappen, and Laurie Herndon, and colleagues in a project supported by the Commonwealth Fund based at Florida Atlantic University. Initial versions of the INTERACT Tools were developed by Dr. Ouslander and colleagues at the Georgia Medical Care Foundation with the support of a special study contract from the Center for Medicare & Medicaid Services. Used with permission.

Figure 5-18. Instructions for Resident Transfer Form and Acute Care Transfer Envelope with Checklist

---

INTERACT

Instructions for Resident Transfer Form

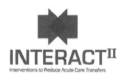

INTERACT^{II}
Interventions to Reduce Acute Care Transfers

Purpose:

This form is completed on every resident who is transferred to the emergency department for evaluation and treatment. The purpose is to provide information about the resident's change in condition, a short narrative about what happened and the reason why the resident is being transferred (e.g., "short of breath, no improvement after 3 days of antibiotics," "fell and now has change in mental status."

Consistent use of this tool will help your nursing home:

- Provide essential information to emergency department staff that will lead to the most appropriate evaluation of your residents
- Insure the safe handoff of your residents to the emergency department

When to complete:

Page 1 of this form should always be completed and sent in the transfer envelope with the resident, since it contains essential information that the emergency department staff may need to make decisions about the resident. Page 2 also contains important information, but may be faxed to the hospital after the resident has been transferred, in the case of a 911 transfer or resident in unstable condition, or it may be sent along with the page 1.

Who to involve:

Generally, the nurse has discussed the transfer with a physician/PA/NP (primary or covering) prior to transfer. It is helpful to include any clinical information from the provider in the Reason for Transfer section. The name of the provider, and how to reach him or her should always be included. The nurse completing the form should sign it, even if another nurse (e.g., a supervisor) is listed as the person to contact for questions about the resident. The staff nurse might complete the form; she should then sign it. The supervisor might be the right person to contact for questions later, if the staff nurse is going home. A Provider to Provider (physician/NP/PA) telephone call is strongly recommended, so that the medical details can be shared among the nursing home and emergency department staff. A nurse to nurse telephone call is also strongly recommended, so that specific nursing issues and changes in resident status can be communicated. Complete the section of the form that asks who made this call and who at the ED received the call. If a resident returns to the nursing home after an emergency department evaluation, a telephone call from the ED nurse to the nursing home nurse is strongly encouraged.

Helpful Hints:

- **Complete all sections of the tool**: The tool is designed to help guide you write a brief but comprehensive summary of the resident's situation.
- **Do not rewrite information that exists elsewhere that is being sent with the resident.** If the SBAR form has been completed, write "see SBAR" for sections with similar information

Figure 5-18. Instructions for Resident Transfer Form and Acute Care Transfer Envelope with Checklist, *continued*

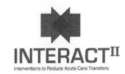

INTERACT *II*

Instructions for Acute Care Transfer Envelope

Purpose:
This checklist (on the outside of the transfer envelope) is completed on every resident who is transferred to the emergency department for evaluation and treatment. The purpose is to provide a single envelope with all the necessary forms inside that the emergency department staff need to evaluate and manage the resident.

Consistent use of this tool will help your nursing home:
- Provide essential information in one, easily recognizable place, to emergency department staff that will lead to the most appropriate evaluation of your residents
- Insure the safe handoff of your residents to the emergency department

When to complete:
Use the checklist to systematically determine that all of the necessary paperwork has been sent with the resident. As each document is placed in the envelope, check off the appropriate box on the outside to indicate that the document has been included.

Who to involve:
The person completing the checklist should sign it and request a signature from the EMS or ambulance personnel who accept the envelope, indicating that all required documents have been sent.

These instructions provide additional detail on proper use of the Resident Transfer Form (Figure 5-16, pages 107–108) and the Acute Care Transfer Envelope with Checklist (Figure 5-17, page 109).

Source: © 2010 Florida Atlantic University. The INTERACT II Tools, educational materials, and implementation strategies were developed by Drs. Joseph Ouslander, Gerri Lamb, Alice Bonner, and Ruth Tappen, and Laurie Herndon, and colleagues in a project supported by the Commonwealth Fund based at Florida Atlantic University. Initial versions of the INTERACT Tools were developed by Dr. Ouslander and colleagues at the Georgia Medical Care Foundation with the support of a special study contract from the Center for Medicare & Medicaid Services. Used with permission.

improve the quality of home health care. The goals of the campaign are to reduce hospital admissions and to help patients better manage their home medications.[38]

Each month, home health leaders develop a new Best Practice Intervention Package that home health agencies can use to help educate staff about interventions that may reduce hospitalizations for home health patients or help them better manage their medications.[38]

The Home Health Quality Improvement Campaign's Transitional Care Coordination Package includes the following tools[38]:

- Quick Tips for Talking with Your Doctor
- Monthly Best Practice Intervention Package Poster
- Personal Health Record Booklet
- Discharge Criteria and Face Sheet (*see* Figure 5-19, pages 112–113)
- Electronic Post-Tests
- Transitional Care Coordination for Clinicians (Podcast)
- Transitional Care Coordination for Medical Social Workers and Home Health Aides (Podcast)
- Educational WebEx

Figure 5-19. Discharge Criteria and Face Sheet

Discharge Criteria

Acceptable Discharge
(Check all applicable)

Independent in ADLs_____
Competent/dependable
    caregivers in the home_____
Lives alone with generous
    support_____
Stable chronic disease_____
Mentally/cognitively alert_____
Compliant with instructions_____

Discharge to retirement home/Assisted living
Appropriate
Discharge to home health – *Complete face sheet*

Review with patient BEFORE discharge
(Check all applicable)

DNR _____
Advance directive _____
Mental health resources_____
MSW involvement _____
PT, OT, ST _____
Nursing _____
Pharmaceutical review of meds _____
Durable medical equipment education_____
Oxygen company notified before discharge_____
Medicaid/office of public assistance_____
Medicaid Personal Assistance Program_____
Medicaid Self Direct PAS Program _____
HCBS Waiver Program case management_____
Social Security _____
Noncompliance contract/consequence_____
Literacy program education _____
Cultural barriers _____
Personal health record_____

Use Caution
Before Discharge
(Check all applicable)

Psychological issues _____
No competent/dependable
    Caregiver_____
Low literacy_____
Lives alone _____
9 or more medications _____
Oxygen therapy _____
ADL assistance_____
Transfer_____
Ambulation _____
PT_____ OT_____ ST_____
Pressure ulcers _____
TPN _____
IV _____

Swing bed, personal care home and nursing home
Appropriate
Discharge to Home Health - *Complete face sheet*

HIGH RISK FOR HOSPITALIZATION!
Patient Education/disease specific _____
Hospice Education _____
Medication management _____
Caregiver education _____

High Risk
(Check applicable)
6 or more indicate high risk for
emergent care

Help with managing meds _____
Discharged from a hospital or SNF _____
Hospitalizations/ER past 12 months _____
Neoplasm as primary diagnosis _____
No competent/dependable caregiver in home _____
Lives alone _____
History of noncompliance_____ falls _____
ADL needs_____ COPD_____ CHF _____
Diabetes_____ Chronic skin ulcers _____
Open wound(s)_____ Confusion _____
Urinary catheter_____ Dyspnea _____
Poor prognosis_____ Short life expectancy _____
HIV/AIDS _____ >2 Secondary diagnoses _____
New diagnosis_____ Financial concerns or
    low socioeconomic status _____

TOTAL CHECKED_____

Appropriate to discharge to nursing
home & assisted living
Discharge to home health –
Complete face sheet

Patient Name _____
DOB _____
Expected Date of Discharge_____

This material was prepared by Mountain-Pacific Quality Health, the Medicare Quality
Improvement Organization for Montana, Wyoming, Hawaii and Alaska, under contract with the Centers for
Medicare & Medicaid Services (CMS), an agency of the U.S. Department of Health and Human
Services. Contents do not necessarily reflect CMS policy. Page 1 8thSOW-MPQHF-HHQ1-07-06.

(continued on page 113)

Figure 5-19. Discharge Criteria and Face Sheet, *continued*

FACE SHEET – DISCHARGE TO HOME HEALTH

Patient Name_____ Ht:____ Wt:____ Lives Alone (Yes) (No)

Address:_____ City_____ St_____ Zip_____

Diagnosis_____,_____,_____

Physician_____ Contact Name_____

Competent/Dependable Caregiver_____

REQUIRED DOCUMENTATION (Please check)

Medicare A____ Medicare B ____ Medicare D____ Medicaid ____ Private Insurance ____	***If discharging patient over the weekend, send supplies and medication home with patient until home health agency does SOC.	Date of Discharge:____/____/____ Date of Assessment____/____/____ Date of Admission ____/____/____ √ High Risk Referral ____
History & Physical ____ Comments:	Discharge Instruction Sheet ____ Comments:	Patient Education: Cardio Pulmonary ____ Diabetes ____ Oxygen ____ Medication ____ Disease Management ____ Other ____ _____ _____
Consultation Reports ____ Comments:	Discharge Order ____ Comments:	Injectable/Medication Mgmt. TPN Insert Date: ____/____/____ Antibiotics & Medication Physician Orders ____
Pertinent Lab X-Ray & Procedure Reports ____ Comments:	Advanced Directives, Code Status ____ Comments:	Line Care PICC Care/ ____ Specify Size, Type & Insert Date:_____ _____ _____ Other Vascular Access Device: ____ Insert Date:_____
Allergy List ____ Comments:	Nutrition ____ Enternal Feed/PEG/PEJ ____ Insertion Date:____/____/____ Other_____	Wound Care Orders & Instruction Wound Vac ____ Other:_____ ____
PT, OT, ST Evaluations & Restrictions ____ Comments:	Oxygen Therapy ____ Physician Orders ____ Oxygen Provider:	Catheters ____ Foley Size _____ Insert Date ____/____/____
DME ____ Provider Name: _____	Laboratory Home Health to Draw ____ Discharge Lab ____ Orders_____ ____	*Additional Comments:*
Additional Comments:	*Additional Comments:*	

This material was prepared by Mountain-Pacific Quality Health, the Medicare Quality Improvement Organization for Montana, Wyoming, Hawaii and Alaska, under contract with the Centers for Medicare & Medicaid Services (CMS), an agency of the U.S. Department of Health and Human Services. Contents do not necessarily reflect CMS policy. Page 2 8th SOW-MPQHF-HHQI-07-06.

This chart can help caregivers make sure that important information is transferred to the home health agency at discharge.

Source: This information originated with Mountain-Pacific Quality Health, the Medicare Quality Improvement Organization for Montana, Wyoming, Hawaii, and Arkansas, under contract with the U.S. Centers for Medicare & Medicaid Services (CMS), an agency of the U.S. Department of Health & Human Services. This information has been reprinted with permission. Contents do not reflect CMS policy.

References

1. American Academy of Family Physicians (AAFP). *Family Medicine in Hospitals: Strategies for Strength.* Leawood, KS: AAFP, 2004.

2. Borowitz S., et al.: Adequacy of information transferred at resident sign-out (inhospital handover of care): A prospective survey. *Qual Saf Health Care* 17:6–10, Feb. 2008.

3. Horwitz L., et al.: What are covering doctors told about their patients? Analysis of sign-out among internal medicine house staff. *Qual Saf Health Care* 18:248–255, Aug. 2009.

4. Philibert I.: Use of strategies from high-reliability organisations to the patient hand-off by resident physicians: Practical implications. *Qual Saf Health Care* 18:261–266, Aug. 2009.

5. The Joint Commission: *Improving Hand-Off Communication.* Oak Brook, IL: Joint Commission Resources, 2007.

6. Sullivan E.: Hand-off communication. *J Perianesth Nurs* 22:275–279, Aug. 2007.

7. Amato-Vealey E., Barba M., Vealey R.: Hand-off communication: A requisite for perioperative patient safety. *AORN J* 88:763–770, Nov. 2008.

8. Staggers N., Jennings B.: The content and context of change of shift report on medical and surgical units. *J Nurs Adm* 39:393–398, Sep. 2009.

9. Boutilier S.: Leaving critical care: Facilitating a smooth transition. *Dimens Crit Care Nurs* 26:137–142, Jul.–Aug. 2007.

10. Nelson B., Massey R.: Implementing an electronic change-of-shift report using Transforming Care at the Bedside processes and methods. *J Nurs Adm* 40:162–168, Apr. 2010.

11. Berkenstadt H., et al.: Improving handoff communications in critical care: Utilizing simulation-based training toward process improvement in managing patient risk. *Chest* 134:158–162, Jul. 2008.

12. Parker J.: *Patient Safety Week Blogs: Day 3, Handoff Communications.* Joint Commission Resources, Mar. 2009. http://www.jcrinc.com/Blog/2009/3/9/Patient-Safety-Week-Blogs-Day-3-Handoff-Communications/ (accessed Aug. 25, 2010).

13. Walrath J., Dang D., Nyberg D.: Hospital RNs' experiences with disruptive behavior: A qualitative study. *J Nurs Care Qual* 25:105–116, Apr.–Jun. 2010.

14. Johnson C.: Bad blood: Doctor-nurse behavior problems impact patient care. *Physician Exec* 35:6–11, Nov.–Dec. 2009.

15. McFetridge B., et al.: An exploration of the handover process of critically ill patients between nursing staff from the emergency department and the intensive care unit. *Nurs Crit Care* 12:261–269, Nov.–Dec. 2007.

16. Horwitz L., et al.: Dropping the baton: A qualitative analysis of failures during the transition from emergency department to inpatient care. *Ann Emerg Med* 53:701–710, Jun. 2009.

17. Terrell K., Miller D.: Critical review of transitional care between nursing homes and emergency departments. *Ann Longterm Care* 15, Feb. 2007. http://www.annalsoflongtermcare.com/article/6782 (accessed Jul. 19, 2010).

18. National Transitions of Care Coalition (NTOCC): *Improving on Transitions of Care: How to Implement and Evaluate a Plan.* Little Rock, AR: NTOCC, 2008.

19. National Transitions of Care Coalition (NTOCC): *Improving Transitions of Care: The Vision of the National Transitions of Care Coalition.* Little Rock, AR: NTOCC, 2008.

20. LaMantia M., et al.: Interventions to improve transitional care between nursing homes and hospitals: A systematic review. *J Am Geriatr Soc* 58:777–782, Apr. 2010.

21. Drury L.: Transition from hospital to home care: What gets lost between the discharge plan and the real world? *J Contin Educ Nurs* 39:198–199, May 2008.

22. The Joint Commission: *The Pharmacist's Role in Patient Safety.* Oak Brook, IL: Joint Commission Resources, 2007.

23. National Coordinating Council for Medication Error Reporting and Prevention: *Recommendations to Enhance Accuracy of Prescription Writing.* Jun. 2005. http://www.nccmerp.org/council/council1996-09-04.html (accessed Jun. 19, 2010).

24. New York State Department of Health: *Discharge Planning.* Jul. 2010. http://www.health.state.ny.us/professionals/patients/discharge_planning/index.htm (accessed Aug. 25, 2010).

25. National Alliance for Caregiving, United Hospital Fund of New York: *A Family Caregiver's Guide to Hospital Discharge Planning.* http://www.caregiving.org/pubs/brochures/familydischargeplanning.pdf (accessed Jul. 19, 2010).

26. Shank B.: California dreamin': Twenty hospitals will be first to use Project BOOST's tuition-based model. *Hospitalist* 14:6, 8, Jul. 2010.

27. PlainLanguage.gov: *Improving Communication from the Federal Government to the Public (Home Page).* http://www.plainlanguage.gov (accessed Aug. 25, 2010).

28. Joint Commission Resources: Strategies for improving health literacy. *The Joint Commission Perspectives on Patient Safety* 8:8–9, Mar. 2008.

29. Hadjistavropoulos H., et al.: Patient perceptions of hospital discharge: Reliability and validity of a patient continuity of care questionnaire. *Int J Qual Health Care* 20:314–323, Oct. 2008.

30. Cleary M., Walter G., Horsfall J.: Handover in psychiatric settings: Is change needed? *J Psychosoc Nurs Ment Health Serv* 47:28–33, Mar. 2009.

31. Rands G., et al.: How consultation liaison meetings improved staff knowledge, communication and care. *Nurs Times* 105:18–20, Oct.–Nov. 2009.

32. Colón-Emeric C., et al.: Patterns of medical and nursing staff communication in nursing homes: Implications and insights from complexity science. *Qual Health Res* 16:173–188, Feb. 2006.

33. Tjia J., et al.: Nurse-physician communication in the long-term care setting: Perceived barriers and impact on patient safety. *J Patient Saf* 5:145–152, Sep. 2009.

34. Kogan P., et al.: Performance improvement in managed long-term care: Physician communication in managing community-dwelling older adults. *Home Healthc Nurse* 28:105–114, Feb. 2010.

35. INTERACT II: *Working Together to Improve Care and Reduce Acute Care Transfers (Home Page).* 2010. http://interact.geriu.org/ (accessed Aug. 25, 2010).

36. Hohl D.: Transitions in home care. *Home Healthc Nurse* 27:499–502, Sep. 2009.

37. Brown E., et al.: Transition to home care: Quality of mental health, pharmacy, and medical history information. *Int J Psychiatry Med* 36(3):339–349, 2006.

38. Home Health Quality Improvement: *Home Health Quality Improvement National Campaign.* 2010. http://www.homehealthquality.org/hh/default.aspx (accessed Aug. 25, 2010).

Chapter 6

Monitoring and Evaluating Transitions of Care

As with all performance improvement activities, the quality department of an organization typically bears primary responsibility for the development and implementation of a program regarding transitions of care. To succeed, however, the program must have the support of both organization leadership and the staff members who actually participate in the transitions of care. Such support is easier to gain when the organization has a strong patient focus and maintains a culture of safety.

One of the greatest challenges in trying to monitor transitions of care is knowing exactly what type of information should be shared for each specific transition and in how much detail. "Organizations sometimes want a 'one size fits all' approach to communication during transitions of care rather than taking into consideration the reason for the transition; the professionals involved; and the care, treatment, or services to be provided by the receiver of the information," says Jane Schetter, R.N., M.S.N., C.N.S., senior consultant, Joint Commission Resources. "Whether or not the receiver will have an opportunity to review documentation prior to care, as well as the level of care to be provided by the receiving service, may determine the type of information and the depth of communication needed during transitions of care."[1]

Before making changes to your current transition-of-care processes, assess your organization's processes. Is important patient care information already being transferred effectively? Or do you need to revise some of your processes to ensure consistent, effective communication?

When reviewing your current transition-of-care processes, Schetter suggests asking the following questions[2]:
1. What is currently happening during the transition of care?
2. How accurate, complete, and clear is the information being shared?
3. Who is involved in the transition of care?
4. Is there an opportunity for questions?

5. If someone has concerns about information received during a transition of care, is there a process in place for information to be verified?

According to Schetter, when reviewing the various types of transitions of care, the focus should be not only on the process itself but also on the effectiveness of the transition. "Effectiveness can be evaluated by looking at each transition and asking if the receiver can safely provide care, treatment, or services to the patient based on the communication and any supportive documentation that is immediately available," she says.[1]

Start reviewing your current processes by doing an initial inventory. What transition-of-care processes currently exist, and how are they being conducted? After you have determined what transition-of-care processes your organization has in place, analyze your processes by comparing the information that needs to be provided during each transition of care with the information that is actually being provided. If the appropriate information is already being shared, it may be that your organization already has an effective standardized method for communication during transitions of care and your processes do not need to be revised.

Other questions that may help you evaluate your current transition-of-care processes include the following[3]:
- Is there a time lag between admission and clarification of which physician will cover the patient and when?
- Does the nurse know the care plan, so he or she can implement it?
- Do patient belongings get lost between the emergency department and inpatient room?
- Does your phone system cut people off when they are on hold?
- When a patient goes from the reception area in outpatient services to an ancillary testing area, does his or her information go along?

- When the physician makes a medication change, does the change reach pharmacy and nursing in a timely fashion so that no error occurs?
- When a family member calls to send a message to the patient, does the patient receive it consistently?
- When the patient sees the doctor for a review of test results, has the doctor already received the results?
- When a new patient is about to be admitted, is environmental services alerted in time to prepare a clean room in a timely fashion?
- Is the receiving unit notified and ready with a greeter so the patient feels personally welcomed?

If you answered "no" to any of these questions, it may be time to review and revise your transition-of-care processes.

Conducting a Failure Mode and Effects Analysis (FMEA) on Transitions of Care

Failure mode and effects analysis (FMEA) is a team-based, systematic, proactive technique that is used to prevent system and process problems *before* they occur (*see* Sidebar 6-1 for steps in conducting an FMEA). FMEA examines which problems, or *failure modes,* could occur within a particular process, such as a transition of care, and anticipates how severe the effects of such problems could be. FMEA assumes that even when people are highly knowledgeable and skilled, failures will occur in some situations.

When assembling an FMEA team, organizations should consider the knowledge and expertise of the potential team members on the transition of care being studied. The team should be multidisciplinary to ensure that different perspectives or viewpoints are brought to the improvement process, and both the team and the organization's leadership should be committed to performance improvement. The team also should include representatives from areas that may be affected by the changes in a redesigned process. For example, if the organization is studying potential failure modes during nursing shift changes, nurses from each unit being studied should be included on the team.

Organizations also should consider including someone on the team who has some distance from the transition of care being studied to serve as an adviser or facilitator and to provide a fresh perspective. This person could be someone who is not at all familiar with the process or event but who possesses excellent analytic skills.

Sidebar 6-1. Steps for Conducting a Failure Mode and Effects Analysis (FMEA)

1. Select a high-risk process and assemble a team.
2. Diagram the process and brainstorm potential failure modes.
3. Determine the effects of the failure modes.
4. Prioritize the failure modes.
5. Identify root causes of the failure modes.
6. Redesign the process.
7. Analyze and test the new process.
8. Implement and monitor the redesigned process.

Studying Transition-of-Care Processes

To effectively study a transition-of-care process, organizations should diagram, collect data on, and brainstorm about the process and how failures could happen. One effective tool for studying a process is a flowchart, which is a pictorial summary that shows with symbols and words the steps, sequence, and relationship of the various operations involved in the performance of a function or a process. (An example of a flowchart appears later in this chapter as Figure 6-1, page 120.) When diagramming transition-of-care processes, organizations should make sure that their diagrams are constructed with the help of individuals who actually perform the work being charted so that the diagrams represent reality.

Determining Root Causes

After a transition-of-care process has been studied, the FMEA team must determine at what points the process could possibly fail. Then the team must identify the underlying reasons, or root causes, for these potential failures. A *root cause* is a fundamental reason for the failure or inefficiency of a process. *Root cause analysis* is a process for identifying the basic or causal factor(s) underlying variation in performance, including the occurrence or possible occurrence of a sentinel event. Root cause analysis can help identify processes that could benefit from FMEA and can specifically determine the roots of an unidentified problem.

Teams may want to look for causes that relate to the following organizational functions:
- *Leadership:* Is the organization's culture based on teamwork and open communication?
- *Human resources:* Are staff members trained and of sufficient number and expertise?

- *Information management:* Is important and accurate information available when needed?

One organization that conducted a failure mode and effects analysis on its discharge medication reconciliation process found many potential failure points and gaps in its existing process. For example, a major component of the organization's discharge medication reconciliation process was a computerized medication form containing both inpatient and home medication lists. Because computerized prescriber order entry was not available, the medication reconciliation form was printed. One failure mode the organization discovered during the FMEA process was that the form was printing too early, which resulted in forms that were not current at discharge and did not show new medication that had been ordered. In addition, sometimes the form was left in the printer or placed in the wrong patient chart, making it difficult for the physician to locate the form when ready to discharge the patient.[4]

Another failure mode the organization uncovered was that physicians sometimes failed to distinguish between the home and inpatient medication lists. This failure resulted in duplicate medication orders and continuation of some medications that should have been discontinued, such as antibiotics. An additional failure mode was unclear communications with patients about when certain medications were to be discontinued.[4]

Implementing Improvement Initiatives

After a team has identified the root causes of potential communication failures during transitions of care, it must design improvement processes that help address these root causes. The team should brainstorm about these improvement processes and then evaluate and prioritize them so that the most efficient and effective processes are implemented first.

The organization that conducted the FMEA on its discharge medication reconciliation process reviewed the literature and analyzed its results. Then the organization used the information it had gathered to develop a new process. The new discharge medication reconciliation process included the following steps[4]:

1. Print discharge medication reconciliation form on day of discharge.
2. Place form on chart.
3. Physician and registered nurse (RN) together complete and sign form.

4. RN transcribes medications onto the discharge instruction form.
5. RN-to-RN reconciliation is performed with a discharge medication reconciliation form and discharge instruction form.
6. Forward documents to a pharmacist for review.
7. Pharmacist reviews documents and verifies their accuracy.
8. Pharmacist sends verification to unit immediately.
9. RN provides patient with discharge instructions.
10. A phone call follow-up occurs within one to two days.

The flowchart shown in Figure 6-1, page 120, illustrates the new process.

Sample FMEA: Psychosocial Assessments in Behavioral Health Care

The following is a sample FMEA that was conducted on psychosocial assessments in a behavioral health care facility.[5]

Assembling the Team

The team consisted of the director of performance improvement, the coordinator of mental health and case management, and two therapist case managers.

Diagramming the Process, Brainstorming Potential Failure Modes, and Determining the Effects of Failure Modes

The FMEA team used an online outline tool to diagram the process. During the brainstorming process, potential failure modes and possible effects were identified for each step of the process (*see* Table 6-1, page 121).

Prioritizing Failure Modes

When prioritizing failure modes, if team members had difficulty agreeing on a number, they first looked for a compromise. In some cases when a compromise could not be reached, they deferred to the therapist case manager.

Identifying Root Causes of the Failure Modes

In addition to brainstorming, to identify root causes of each potential failure mode, the FMEA team solicited input from other therapist case managers who were not on the FMEA team. Root causes for incomplete or inaccurate transfer of information during transitions of care included client refusal, the receiving caregiver being unavailable when called, computer problems, interruptions, and human error (such as forgetting to call).

Figure 6-1. Discharge Medication Reconciliation

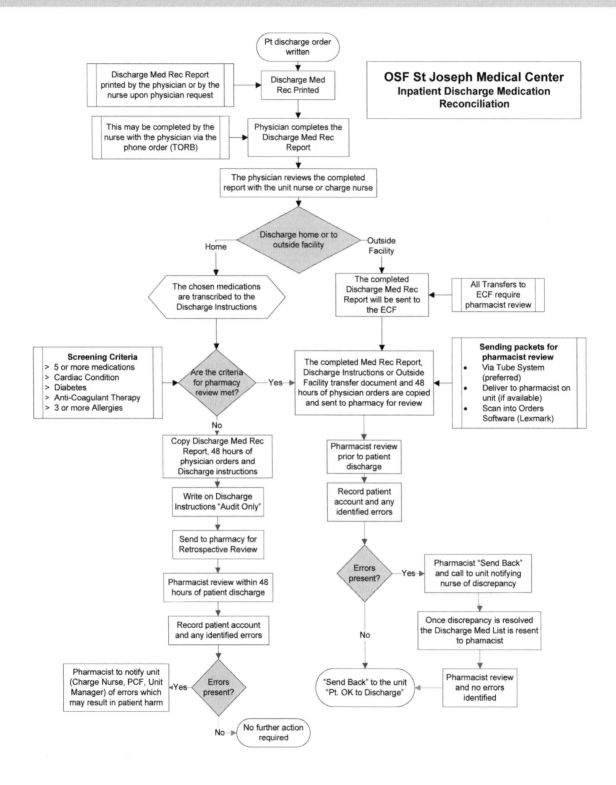

This figure illustrates the steps in the inpatient discharge medication reconciliation process used at OSF St. Joseph Medical Center. The process was developed after the organization conducted a failure mode and effects analysis (FMEA).

Source: OSF St. Joseph Medical Center. Used with permission.

Table 6-1. Steps in the FMEA Process

Step	Failure Mode	Effect
Initial meeting between the client and the therapist takes place.	Client does not show up or leaves before being seen.	A return visit would need to be scheduled.
The initial mental health assessment is completed.	The mental health assessment is not completed.	Treatment cannot be initiated.
Follow-up appointments are scheduled.	Follow-up appointments are not scheduled.	Treatment is delayed.
Client is referred internally to another provider or unit.	Information is not transferred from one provider to the next.	Patient's treatment is delayed or treatment is not appropriate to the patient.
Client is referred externally to another facility.	Information is not transferred from the referring facility or provider to the receiving facility or provider.	Patient's treatment is delayed or treatment is not appropriate to the patient.
Data from the initial encounter form are transferred to the patient record.	The data transferred are incomplete or inaccurate.	Caregivers do not have the information they need to properly treat the patient.

Source: The Joint Commission: *FMEA in Health Care: Proactive Risk Reduction,* 3rd ed. Oak Brook, IL: Joint Commission Resources, 2010.

Redesigning the Process

Because forgetfulness was a major contributor to inadequate transfer of information during transitions of care, the process was redesigned to include prompts or reminders.

Analyzing the New Process

The FMEA team used the Plan-Do-Study-Act reporting form to test new processes as each change was implemented.

Implementing and Monitoring the Redesigned Process

Every quarter, the FMEA team conducts a chart audit and reports back to the performance improvement team.

What to Look for When Monitoring Transition-of-Care Processes

After you have evaluated your current transition-of-care processes and revised them as needed, it is important to continue to monitor those processes to ensure that staff members are fully educated and compliant and to identify any areas that may need additional revision to improve the processes. When monitoring a transition-of-care process, Schetter suggests asking the following questions[2]:

- Which staff members were involved?
- What was the mode of communication?
- What information was provided?
- How timely was the communication?
- Was the information accurate?
- Was the information understood by the person receiving that information? How would the provider of the information know this?
- Was enough information given so that the person receiving the patient could care for him or her safely and effectively?

According to Schetter, organizations should conduct tracers when monitoring transitions of care. "Someone should follow each actual transition of care process and listen to the communication as it takes place," she says. "They should also look at the available documentation, if applicable, and the ability of the receiver to provide care, treatment, or services to the patient based on the communication during the transition of care. Was there a match between the communication provided and the patient's needs?"[1] It is important that staff members remain engaged throughout each transition of care (*see* Sidebar 6-2, page 122).

Another method of monitoring transitions of care is to develop a tool to evaluate the effectiveness of each transition. "Using some type of scale, determine if the transition was effective," Schetter says. "If the organization has an established process for each type of transition of care and the communication required, the scale might include the

Sidebar 6-2. No Automatic Transitions of Care

While monitoring transitions of care, quality improvement specialists at some organizations have noted that staff members are completing the steps in each transition-of-care process without really thinking about what they are doing. Because transitions of care are conducted so frequently, it is easy to see how they could become routine or automatic. However, it is important that staff members stay fully aware of what they are doing during every transition. The following strategies help ensure that staff members actively participate in transitions of care:

- Have someone who is not involved in a case come in for a last-minute check. For example, a staff member from a different department can come in and observe the process.
- Engage a nonclinician, such as an environmental care worker, in the process. Rotate these observers on a regular basis to discourage complacency.
- Consider using a tool, such as Situation–Background–Assessment–Recommendation (SBAR), that forces staff to think about a desired outcome or make a recommendation.
- Rearrange your current forms or checklists so that the eyes are drawn to important data.
- Minimize open-ended responses. Use checklists when feasible.
- Vary the order of checklists to keep them more interesting.

Source: Are handoffs too "automatic"? QI experts fear errors could rise. *Healthcare Benchmarks Qual Improv* 13:1–4, Jan. 2006.

elements of the process and a simple 'yes' or 'no' as to whether or not the information was communicated during the transition. Another method might be to list the information shared during the transition of care and then use a form or scale to confirm whether or not the information shared was accurate."[1]

An example of a tool used for monitoring transitions of care is shown in Figure 6-2, page 123. It is called the Patient Hand-Off Communication Assessment Tool, which was developed by Joint Commission Resources for its Continuous Service Readiness (CSR®) program.

The Care Transitions Measure

The Care Transitions Measure™ is a patient questionnaire used to measure staff performance during the transition from hospital to home. It was designed by Eric A. Coleman, M.D., and colleagues with support from the Commonwealth Fund, the Robert Wood Johnson Foundation, and the Paul Beeson Faculty Scholars in Aging.[6]

The Care Transitions Measure asks a series of questions about how well patients understand their diagnoses, the management of their conditions, their medications, and their follow-up appointments. It has been shown to be not only consistent and reliable but also applicable to multiple facility types. Additionally, the Care Transitions Measure allows organizations to compare responses about discharge preparation between patients who experienced a return visit to the emergency

department or a readmission and those who did not.[6] The questionnaire is available online in English, Spanish, French, Russian, Finnish, Arabic, and Hebrew through the Care Transitions Program Web site (http://www.caretransitions.org/).

Dr. Coleman and colleagues conducted a study[7] to determine whether the Care Transitions Measure could help organizations identify deficiencies in care, use the identified deficiencies to develop a quality improvement program, and determine if the quality improvement program was improving patient care, and to establish whether the specific Care Transitions Measure called CTM-3 could predict return visits to the emergency department. The study was divided into two groups. The purpose of the first group was to establish baseline Care Transitions Measure scores and determine deficiencies in care. Members of the second group—patients with a diagnosis of diabetes or congestive heart failure who were being discharged from the hospital—were recipients of the interventions developed by the hospital as part of the quality improvement program.[7]

As a result of the baseline Care Transitions Measure scores, the hospital developed the following interventions[7]:

- In-services on teamwork and patient-centered care
- Patient education materials aimed at helping patients identify warning signs that may indicate a decline in their condition and to know when, where, and how to seek additional treatment
- Self-management training for both patients and caregivers

Figure 6-2. Patient Hand-Off Communication Assessment Tool

Patient Hand-Off Communication Assessment Tool

The Hand Off situation:		
Staff involved in Hand Off	**Services/Dept/Area of Source**	**Services/Dept/Area of Receiver**
Physician to Physician		
Physician to Nurse		
Physician to *Clinician		
Nurse to Physician		
Nurse to Nurse		
Nurse to Other Clinician		
Clinician to Physician		
Clinician to Nurse		
Clinician to Clinician		
To a non-clinician		
Mode of Communication	Electronic MR☐ Written ☐ Verbal ☐ Audio/tape☐ Other ☐	
Describe		
Special Technique/Form		

Information Provided	Yes	No	N/A	Comment(s)
Diagnosis				
Current condition, any recent changes				
Current treatment, and recent changes				
What to watch for in next interval of care				
Medications				
Precautions (fall, pressure ulcer, etc.)				
Services/disciplines involved				
Code Status/Advance Directives				
Patient's understanding of Dx & Tx				
Special cultural, language or communication needs or considerations.				

Timeliness of Communication:	# of minutes	
From decision to hand off to the hand off communication		
From hand off communication to receiving the patient		
Length of time to share hand off information		

Risk Assessment of Process: Scale 0-5 effectiveness of hand off (score 5 best practice)

	00	01	02	03	04	05	N/A	
Interactive								
Opportunity for questioning								
Interruption limited								
Verification of information								
Review of relevant historical data								
Timeliness of Communication								
Length of time for communication								
Observe care provided to the patient or interview patient for consistency with the information								
Was care needed consistent with the information provided in the hand-off communication								
Goal is to move scores for all applicable areas to best practice.								

*Clinician is any clinician/caregiver other than physician or nurse

This tool can be used to monitor transitions of care.

- Improved accessibility of the patient's discharge plan to all caregivers through the health care system's electronic records

Following implementation of the quality improvement program, Care Transitions Measure scores initially increased significantly over the first three months. However, they then began to decline due to extenuating circumstances (a rumor that the hospital was in financial trouble and reassignment of nurses to different wards).[7] The study also demonstrated that the quality of transitions of care at discharge, as determined by CTM-3 scores, was a significant predictor of emergency department returns within 30 days of discharge.[7]

Online extras

For a link to the Care Transitions Measure, visit http://www.jcrinc.com/HCTC10/Extras/.

Performance Improvement Methodologies

The Joint Commission Center for Transforming Healthcare recognizes the applicability of certain general performance improvement methodologies in addressing communication during transitions of care. Robust Process Improvement™ (RPI), a problem-solving methodology developed by The Joint Commission, uses a variety of tools to discover specific risk points and contributing factors and then to develop and implement solutions that will improve the effectiveness of communication during transitions of care.

RPI is a set of strategies, tools, methods, and training programs adopted by The Joint Commission for improving its business processes. Application of RPI increases the efficiency of business processes and the quality of The Joint Commission's products and services. A robust process is a process that consistently achieves high quality by doing the following:

- Recognizing and seeking the voice of the customer
- Defining factors critical to quality
- Using data and data analysis to design improvement
- Enlisting stakeholders and process owners in creating and sustaining solutions
- Eliminating defects and waste
- Drastically decreasing failure rates
- Simplifying and increasing the speed of processes
- Partnering with staff and leaders to seek, commit to, and accept change

The RPI toolkit includes methodologies that have been proven effective in many sectors, including health care, and have been used to achieve dramatic improvements in quality and in cost. These methodologies include Lean Six Sigma, Work Out, and formal change management methods. Lean Six Sigma and Work Out produce the best technical solutions. In addition, all the tools in the RPI toolkit have strong philosophical underpinnings that drive and sustain change, such as the value of an empowered work force, the desire for efficiency, and the goal of excellence.

Lean Six Sigma, Work Out, and change management are the basic "tool sets" within RPI. These methodologies have long, illustrious histories, each with supporters and detractors. The phrase *Robust Process Improvement* was coined because The Joint Commission recognized the richness of each of these tool sets and the advantage of a variety of approaches. Each of the tool sets is explained in detail in the following pages.

One of the many strengths of RPI is the combination of technical proficiency in data-driven problem solving (through Lean Six Sigma and Work Out) with the multiplier effect of formal change management processes. The inclusion of change management recognizes that a great technical solution is often not enough for sustainability. Recognizing the needs and ideas of people who are part of a process—and who are charged with implementing a new solution—is important in building acceptance and accountability.

Six Sigma

Six Sigma is a statistical model that measures a process in terms of defects. Six Sigma enables an organization to achieve quality by using a set of strategies, tools, and methods designed to improve processes so that less than 3.4 defects (errors) exist per million opportunities, and processes are as near to perfect as possible. Sigma, or the Greek letter δ, is the symbol for standard deviation in statistics. Standard deviation levels help us understand how much the process deviates from perfection.

Six Sigma is also a philosophy of management that emphasizes the following:

- The importance of understanding factors critical to quality and customer expectations
- The measurement and analysis of data
- The implementation of solutions designed to improve processes to affect the most statistically significant sources of variation
- Sustaining these solutions

In short, Six Sigma is several things:

- A statistical basis of measurement that strives for reduction of defects to 3.4 defects per million opportunities
- A philosophy and a goal: as perfect as practically possible methodology
- A symbol of quality

Motorola started using Six Sigma in the 1980s to improve its manufacturing processes. General Electric (GE) and other companies expanded its applicability to service processes with great success. Other users and innovators in the late 1990s included DuPont, Dow Chemical, 3M, Ford, Amex, Bank of America, JP Morgan Chase, and United Health Care.[8]

DMAIC (pronounced *duh-MAY-ick*) is an acronym for *Define, Measure, Analyze, Improve,* and *Control.* It is the core of Six Sigma methodology and describes its problem-solving sequence.

- *Define* the work to be done and what is critical to quality from the point of view of the sponsor, customer, and stakeholders.
- *Measure* the baseline performance or competitive current state.
- *Analyze* what we need to do differently by identifying the elements that most significantly affect the variability of a process.
- *Improve* the current state by designing interventions that directly address the most significant sources of variation (identified in the Analyze phase).
- *Control* the process for sustained gains.

Lean

Lean is a well-defined set of tools that increase customer value by eliminating *waste* (also known by the Japanese term *muda*)—that is, any activity that uses resources but provides no value for the customer—and creating flow throughout the value stream. Lean improvements have the following characteristics:

- Are inexpensive to implement
- Focus on improving the process, not the people
- Address the batch-and-queue mentality of silos by following process flow
- Promote simple, error-proof systems

Therefore, a lean process is better (no defects; it is what the customer wants), cheaper (non-value-added work is removed, there is no rework or scrap), and faster (eliminates batch and queue, introduces flow, gets it right the first time).

Lean methodology includes the following steps:

1. *Specify value*—from the customer's perspective.
2. *Map the process* using a process map or value stream map.
3. *Identify value-added and non-value-added steps* in the process.
4. *Examine flow*—for example, continuous, minimally interrupted flow; single piece versus batching.
5. *Create "pull"*—that is, do not produce until the next step downstream is ready for you.
6. *Pursue perfection*—sustain improvement; change culture.

Lean Six Sigma

Recognizing the complementary nature of the two methodologies, many companies have used Lean and Six Sigma concurrently, utilizing different pieces of each tool set to address specific improvement problems along a value stream. This practice of combining different tool sets and playing to strengths is sometimes called the *blended approach.* The Joint Commission's blended approach includes Lean Six Sigma as well as Work Out and the Change Acceleration Process (CAP).

Work Out

Work Out is a structured, systematic way to bring people together to develop rapid, lasting improvements in process performance. The improvements are typically implemented in 90 to 120 days. Former GE CEO Jack Welch observed, "Trust the people in the organization—the people in the best position to improve a business are the people in the job every day."[9] This reflection goes to the heart of what makes Work Out so powerful. By design it engages the best thinking from those in the organization who are closest to the processes, who "live them" daily and who invariably have many ideas for improvement.

A Work Out starts by setting a specific, measurable challenge and goal, by identifying the cross-functional set of participants who need to be involved, and by collecting relevant data prior to the Work Out event. Although planning and preparation usually take four to six weeks and implementation occurs over 90 days, the Work Out event itself takes only one day.[9]

Change Management

The Joint Commission uses formal change management methods that are a set of actions, supported by a tool set, used to prepare an organization to seek, commit to, and accept change. Change management methods increase the exposure and participation of staff and leadership in shaping new solutions and interventions. Change management tools increase the speed in which the proposed change is adapted and accepted, and they reinforce its effectiveness.

The Joint Commission uses the Change Acceleration Process (CAP) model of change management developed by General Electric. CAP was created by GE to facilitate employees' ability to improve processes by engaging them in managing the constant change that is inherent in any dynamic business environment.

The following seven phases of CAP describe what is necessary for an organization to most effectively make the transition from its current state to the desired improved state:
1. Leading change
2. Creating a shared need

3. Shaping a vision
4. Mobilizing commitment
5. Making change last
6. Monitoring progress
7. Changing systems and structures

The Joint Commission trains staff in RPI methods. RPI methods are becoming part of the daily work of The Joint Commission and are being used to increase the organization's capacity for improvement. RPI methods are also used by The Joint Commission Center for Transforming Healthcare in creating durable solutions to persistent health care problems. Members of health care organizations who participate in Center improvement projects have in-house expertise in RPI.

References

1. Jane Schetter, e-mail message to Julie Henry, Mar. 28, 2010.
2. The Joint Commission: *Improving Hand-Off Communication.* Oak Brook, IL: Joint Commission Resources, 2007.
3. Leebov W.: The connective tissue issue. *Hosp Health Netw,* Aug. 2006. http://www.hhnmag.com/hhnmag_app/jsp/articledisplay.jsp?dcrpath=HHNMAG/PubsNewsArticle/data/2006August/060815HHN_Online_Leebov&domain=HHNMAG (accessed Aug. 25, 2010).
4. Joint Commission Resources: Using six sigma methodologies: Creating a revised discharge medication reconciliation process. *The Joint Commission Perspectives on Patient Safety* 10:1, 3–6, Jan. 2010.
5. The Joint Commission: *FMEA in Health Care: Proactive Risk Reduction,* 3rd ed. Oak Brook, IL: Joint Commission Resources, 2010.
6. The Care Transitions Program. *The Care Transitions Measure.* http://www.caretransitions.org/ctm_main.asp (accessed Aug. 25, 2010).
7. Coleman E. (ed.): The central role of performance measurement in improving the quality of transitional care. In *Charting a Course for High Quality Care Transitions.* Binghamton, NY: Haworth Press, 2007, pp. 93–104.
8. Brue G.: *Six Sigma for Managers.* New York City: McGraw-Hill, 2002.
9. Harris D.: *Work Out: The Most Powerful Process Improvement Tool.* Aug. 27, 2007. http://www.isixsigma.com/index.php?option=com_k2&view=item&id=313:work-out-the-most-powerful-process-improvement-tool&Itemid=181 (accessed Aug. 25, 2010).

Chapter 7

Case Studies on Transitions of Care

Many organizations have developed initiatives to improve communication during transitions of care. This chapter examines some of those initiatives in detail. Available tools, forms, or checklists are provided.

CASE STUDY: PROJECT RED

To improve the quality of the organization's discharge process, a team from Boston Medical Center developed Project RED (Re-Engineered Discharge), a tool designed to improve work-flow processes and reduce readmission rates. The goal of Project RED is to improve patient safety by helping patients better understand their diagnoses, treatments, and medications, and to help them schedule their follow-up visits. The Project RED initiative is based on 11 components (*see* Sidebar 7-1).

When preparing a patient for discharge under the Project RED initiative, a nurse enters specific patient information into a computer template. The data are then compiled electronically into a booklet called the After Hospital Care Plan (*see* Figure 7-1, page 128). The After Hospital Care Plan includes the following[1]:

- Diagnosis
- Medications (name of medication, when to take the medication, reason for taking the medication, how much medication to take, and how to take the medication)
- Follow-up appointments
- Educational materials about the patient's condition
- Provider contact information

The After Hospital Care Plan is written in simple language. To ensure patient understanding, a virtual patient advocate or a nurse reviews the After Hospital Care Plan with the patient and also schedules any follow-up visits. If they wish, patients may choose to receive their discharge instructions from a "virtual nurse" named Louise via computer (*see* Figure 7-2,

Sidebar 7-1. Components of Project RED
1. Educate the patient about his or her condition during the time in the hospital.
2. Use patient input to make postdischarge appointments.
3. Inform patient of in-hospital tests and follow up on results.
4. Organize postdischarge services.
5. Explain and discuss the medication plan.
6. Reconcile the discharge plan with national guidelines and critical pathways.
7. Review the appropriate information and steps in case a problem arises.
8. Quickly relay the discharge summary to the postdischarge medical personnel.
9. Ask the patient to explain the care plan in his or her own words.
10. Give the patient a written plan at the time of discharge.
11. Follow up by phone shortly after discharge.

page 128). The empathetic virtual nurse guides patients through the process and allows them to ask questions using a touch screen. If there are any issues that Louise cannot resolve, they are then addressed by a live nurse.

To help prevent adverse drug events, a pharmacist calls the patient a few days after discharge to check on the patient's progress.[1] In addition, the pharmacist assesses whether the

Figure 7-1. After Hospital Care Plan

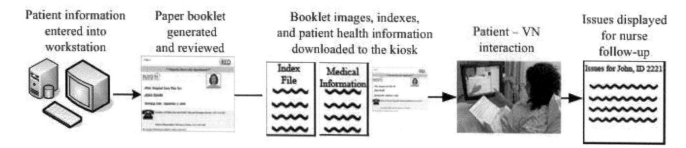

Patient information entered into workstation → Paper booklet generated and reviewed → Booklet images, indexes, and patient health information downloaded to the kiosk → Patient – VN interaction → Issues displayed for nurse follow-up

This flowchart depicts the steps nurses follow as part of a patient's discharge as part of Project RED.

Source: Boston Medical Center. Used with permission.

Figure 7-2. Louise, a Virtual Nurse

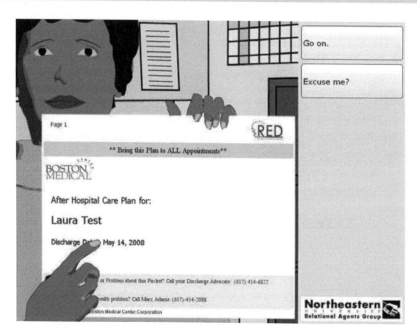

Louise guides patients through discharge instructions and allows them to ask questions until the instructions are clear.

Source: Boston Medical Center. Used with permission.

patient has obtained all medications and if he or she is using the After Hospital Care Plan and taking medications as directed. The importance of going to all follow-up appointments is again reinforced, and patients are instructed to bring the After Hospital Care Plan to each appointment.

Evaluation

The RED intervention was compared to standard discharge procedures, and the results were published in the *Annals of Internal Medicine* in early 2009. The study showed that the RED intervention prevented one-third of postdischarge hospital readmissions and eliminated one emergency department visit for every 7.3 patients. Additionally, 94% of the RED intervention patients were discharged from the hospital with a scheduled follow-up appointment; only 35% in the control group were discharged with a scheduled appointment for follow-up.[2]

Further Information

For more information on Project RED, go online to http://www.bu.edu/fammed/projectred/index.html.

CASE STUDY: PROJECT **BOOST**

On July 10, 2008, the Philadelphia-based Society of Hospital Medicine (SHM) launched Project BOOST (Better Outcomes for Older adults through Safe Transitions). The purpose of this initiative is to improve the care of older patients as they make the transition from hospital to home.[3]

Project BOOST was developed by leading hospitalists and the Society of Hospital Medicine with guidance from a national advisory board chaired by Eric Coleman, M.D., M.P.H. The board was established in an effort to create a national consensus for best practices. It includes representatives from the U.S. Centers for Medicare & Medicaid Services, the Agency for Healthcare Research and Quality, The Joint Commission, and Blue Cross and Blue Shield Association, along with specialists in geriatrics, nursing, pharmacy, patient advocacy, and other fields. Project BOOST's principal investigator, Mark V. Williams, M.D., F.H.M., received input from experienced hospitalists with expertise in transitions of care and quality improvement, including the following:

- Jeff Greenwald, M.D., S.F.H.M.
- Eric Howell, M.D., S.F.H.M.
- Greg Maynard, M.D., M.S., S.F.H.M.
- Lakshmi Halasyamani, M.D., S.F.H.M.
- Arpana Vidyarthi, M.D., F.H.M.

"Project BOOST offers a proven opportunity for hospitals and health care teams to improve patient safety at the point of hospital discharge and reduce readmissions," says Dr. Williams.[4]

Project BOOST utilizes a team approach to assess patients' risk for rehospitalization and provides risk-specific discharge planning activities to optimize the hospital discharge transition. Initial development of Project BOOST was funded by the John A. Hartford Foundation. "SHM has a long-standing relationship with The John A. Hartford Foundation," says Tina Budnitz, M.P.H., senior advisor, Society of Hospital Medicine. "We started the project by working with them to examine what people are doing around the country, identify the 'make or break' interventions being used by the best and brightest, and develop the clinical and project management tools needed to fill any existing gaps."[5]

The project comprises three major elements[3]:

1. **A discharge planning toolkit**
    -   The toolkit includes evidence- and expert-based interventions for risk assessment, discharge education utilizing teach-back processes, and guidance for determining the need, timing, and content of follow-up communications with receiving physicians, patients, and families.
    -   The toolkit provides practical resources such as clinical and project management tools (for examples, *see* Figures 7-3 and 7-4, pages 130–131 and 132, respectively); a step-by-step guide to plan, implement, evaluate, and manage the intervention; staff training materials; patient education materials; and a review of key literature.
    -   The entire project toolkit is available online at http://www.hospitalmedicine.org/BOOST.

2. **Training and technical support for sites implementing the toolkit**
    -   A yearlong mentoring program that includes six components:
        1. A 2-day training session for the improvement team
        2. Scheduled calls between team leaders and mentor(s)
        3. Individualized support using the BOOST toolkit for improvement
        4. A Web-based peer collaboration network that includes a Web-based clinical database for benchmarking, a Listserv™, and document sharing
        5. A DVD and companion curriculum for nurse educators to train nurses on how to use the teach-back process
        6. A site visit from a mentor who meets with team members and senior leaders (for example, the chief executive officer, the chief nursing officer, and/or the chief medical officer) and can present at a hospital's grand rounds
    -   Daylong precourses at Society of Hospital Medicine annual meetings
    -   Webinars related to improving the discharge process
    -   An Online Care Transitions Resource Room containing the toolkit, an implementation guide, and access to online discussion forums with leading experts. The resource room can be accessed at http://www.hospitalmedicine.org/BOOST.

3. **Advocacy at the national level to make system changes that support safe transition practices**
    -   Williams served as co-chair of the Physician Consortium for Performance Improvement Committee to establish measurable, meaningful

Figure 7-3. Tool for Addressing Risk: A Geriatric Evaluation for Transitions (TARGET)

Risk Assessment: 7P Screening Tool (Check all that apply.)	Risk Specific Intervention	Signature of individual responsible for insuring intervention administered
Problem medications (anticoagulants, insulin, aspirin & clopidogrel dual therapy, digoxin, narcotics) ☐	☐ Medication specific education using Teach Back provided to patient and caregiver ☐ Monitoring plan developed and communicated to patient and aftercare providers, where relevant (e.g. warfarin, digoxin and insulin) ☐ Specific strategies for managing adverse drug events reviewed with patient/caregiver ☐ Follow-up phone call at 72 hours to assess adherence and complications	
Punk (depression) (screen positive or diagnosis) ☐	☐ Assessment of need for psychiatric aftercare if not in place ☐ Communication with aftercare providers, highlighting this issue if new ☐ Involvement/awareness of support network insured	
Principal diagnosis (cancer, stroke, DM, COPD, heart failure) ☐	☐ Review of national discharge guidelines, where available (e.g. CHF) ☐ Disease specific education using Teach-Back with patient/caregiver ☐ Action plan reviewed with patient/caregivers regarding what to do and who to contact in the event of worsening or new symptoms ☐ Discuss goals of care and chronic illness model discussed with patient/caregiver	
Polypharmacy (≥5 more routine meds) ☐	☐ Elimination of unnecessary medications ☐ Simplification of medication scheduling to improve adherence ☐ Follow-up phone call at 72 hours to assess adherence and complications	
Poor health literacy (inability to do Teach Back) ☐	☐ Committed caregiver involved in planning/administration of all general and risk specific interventions ☐ Aftercare plan education using Teach-Back provided to patient and caregiver ☐ Link to community resources for additional patient/caregiver support ☐ Follow-up phone call at 72 hours to assess adherence and complications	
Patient support (absence of care giver to assist with discharge and home care) ☐	☐ Follow-up phone call at 72 hours to assess condition, adherence and complications ☐ Follow-up appointment with aftercare medical provider within 7 days ☐ Involvement of home care providers of services with clear communications of discharge plan to those providers	
Prior hospitalization (non-elective; in last 6 months) ☐	☐ Review reasons for re-hospitalization in context of prior hospitalization ☐ Follow-up phone call at 72 hours to assess condition, adherence and complications ☐ Follow-up appointment with aftercare medical provider within 7 days	

Complete TARGET by insuring the Universal Patient Discharge Checklist is completed for all patients.

(continued on page 131)

Figure 7-3. Tool for Addressing Risk: A Geriatric Evaluation for Transitions (TARGET), *continued*

Universal Patient Discharge Checklist

		Initials
1.	GAP assessment (see below) completed with issues addressed.............. YES ☐ NO ☐	_____
2.	Medications reconciled with pre-admission list........................... YES ☐ NO ☐	_____
3.	Medication use/side effects reviewed using Teach-Back with patient/caregiver(s)........... YES ☐ NO ☐	_____
4.	Teach-Back used to confirm patient/caregiver understanding of disease, prognosis and self-care requirements................. YES ☐ NO ☐	_____
5.	Action plan for management of symptoms/side effects/complications requiring medical attention established and shared with patient/caregiver using Teach-Back............ YES ☐ NO ☐	_____
6.	Discharge plan (including educational materials; medication list with reason for use and highlighted new/changed/discontinued drugs; follow-up plans) taught and provided to patient/caregiver at discharge................ YES ☐ NO ☐	_____
7.	Discharge communication provided to principal care provider(s)................. YES ☐ NO ☐	_____
8.	Documented receipt of discharge information from principal care provider(s).......... YES ☐ NO ☐	_____
9.	Arrangements made for outpatient follow-up with principal care provider(s)........... YES ☐ NO ☐	_____
	For increased risk patients, consider.............. Not applicable ☐	
1.	Face-to-face multidisciplinary rounds prior to discharge............ YES ☐ NO ☐	_____
2.	Direct communication with principal care provider *before* discharge.......... YES ☐ NO ☐	_____
3.	Phone contact with patient/caregiver arranged within 72 hours post-discharge to assess condition, discharge plan comprehension and adherence, and to reinforce follow-up...... YES ☐ NO ☐	_____
4.	Follow-up appointment with principal care provider within 7 days of discharge............ YES ☐ NO ☐	_____
5.	Direct contact information for hospital personnel familiar with patient's course provided to patient/caregiver to address questions/concerns *if unable to reach principal care provider* prior to first follow-up........... YES ☐ NO ☐	_____

Confirmed by: _____   _____   _____   ___/___/___
                  Signature   Print Name   Date

General Assessment of Preparedness (GAP)

Prior to discharge, evaluate the following areas with the patient/caregiver(s) and ambulatory medical care providers: A = Beginning upon admission; P = Prior to discharge; D = At discharge

Logistical Issues

1.	Functional status assessment completed (P)	YES ☐	NO ☐	N/A ☐
2.	Access (e.g. keys) to home insured (P)	YES ☐	NO ☐	N/A ☐
3.	Home prepared for patient's arrival (P) (e.g. medical equipment, safety evaluation, food)	YES ☐	NO ☐	N/A ☐
4.	Financial resources for care needs assessed (P)	YES ☐	NO ☐	N/A ☐
5.	Ability to obtain medications confirmed (P)	YES ☐	NO ☐	N/A ☐
6.	Responsible party for insuring med adherence identified/prepared, if not patient (P)	YES ☐	NO ☐	N/A ☐
7.	Transportation to initial follow-up arranged (D)	YES ☐	NO ☐	N/A ☐
8.	Transportation home arranged (D)	YES ☐	NO ☐	N/A ☐

Psychosocial Issues

1.	Substance abuse/dependence evaluated (A)	YES ☐	NO ☐	N/A ☐
2.	Abuse/neglect presence assessed (A)	YES ☐	NO ☐	N/A ☐
3.	Cognitive status assessed (A)	YES ☐	NO ☐	N/A ☐
4.	Advanced care planning documented (A)	YES ☐	NO ☐	N/A ☐
5.	Support circle for patient identified (P)	YES ☐	NO ☐	N/A ☐
6.	Contact information for home caregivers obtained and provided to patient (D)	YES ☐	NO ☐	N/A ☐

Confirmed by: _____   _____   ___/___/___
                  Signature   Print Name   Date

This tool, part of the Project BOOST toolkit, helps in risk assessment for older patients.

Source: Jeffrey Greenwald, M.D., S.F.H.M, and Mark V. Williams, M.D., F.A.C.P., F.H.M, Project BOOST in collaboration with The The Society of Hospital Medicine. Used with permission.

Figure 7-4. Patient PASS: Patient Preparation to Address Situations (after discharge) Successfully

I was in the hospital because

If I have the following problems …   I should …

1. _____   1. _____
2. _____   2. _____
3. _____   3. _____
4. _____   4. _____
5. _____   5. _____

Important contact information:

1. My primary doctor: _____
( ) 2. My hospital doctor: _____
( ) 3. My visiting nurse: _____
( ) 4. My pharmacy: _____
( ) 5. Other: _____

I understand my treatment plan. I feel able and willing to participate actively in my care:

_____
Patient/Caregiver Signature

_____
Provider Signature

___/___/___
Date

My appointments:

1. On: __/__/__ at __:__ am/pm For: _____
2. On: __/__/__ at __:__ am/pm For: _____
3. On: __/__/__ at __:__ am/pm For: _____
4. On: __/__/__ at __:__ am/pm For: _____

Tests and issues I need to talk with my doctor(s) about at my clinic visit:

1. _____
2. _____
3. _____
4. _____
5. _____

Other instructions: 1. _____
2. _____
3. _____

This tool, part of the Project BOOST toolkit, helps patients plan their postdischarge follow-up.

Source: Jeffrey Greenwald, M.D., S.F.H.M. and Mark V. Williams, M.D., F.A.C.P., F.H.M., Project BOOST in collaboration with The Society of Hospital Medicine. Used with permission.

performance measures for transitions of care, and he served on technical expert panels on transitions of care for MedPAC and the U.S. Centers for Medicare & Medicaid Services.

- Participation in national consortium efforts to establish principles and standards for health care teams relating to transitions of care. The principles and standards were published in the *Journal of Hospital Medicine*[6] and the *Journal of General Internal Medicine*[7] in 2009.

Implementation

Project BOOST began with 6 pilot sites in 2008 and has now grown to 30 sites that are currently receiving mentoring. Beginning in May 2010, 15 new sites were expected to participate in Project BOOST as part of a Michigan collaborative with the University of Michigan funded by Blue Cross and Blue Shield. In October 2010, 20 sites were scheduled to participate as part of a California regional collaborative supported in part by the California Healthcare Foundation. "There is tremendous enthusiasm for this project," Budnitz says. "We're delighted to see the project have such tremendous spread and reach with both national and regional collaboratives."[5]

Evaluation

A number of methods are being used to evaluate Project BOOST. "First there's the technical support aspect, which we're evaluating through qualitative interviews with the sites," Budnitz says. "We're also collecting global metrics from the participating sites, such as 30-day all-cause readmission rates, length of stay, patient satisfaction scores, and communication between discharging and receiving physicians. Sites have varied demographics and include academic and community

settings, urban and rural settings, and small and large facilities. Preliminary data from the pilot sites indicates that they have started to see a decrease in all 30-day all-cause readmission rates and an increase in patient satisfaction scores."[5] About 18,000 patient discharges have been impacted by Project BOOST interventions.[3]

online extras

For a link to the entire Project BOOST toolkit, visit http://www.jcrinc.com/HCTC10/Extras/.

"What's unique about this approach is the philosophy that you have to look at change at the system level," Budnitz says. "When you impart these types of skills to a hospital team, they will be able to use them for other quality improvement projects as well. So at the same time we're improving patient safety at the time of discharge, we're building capacity within the clinical team to address any number of quality issues. It's like the difference between giving someone a fishing lesson versus just a fishing rod."[5]

Open enrollment for Project Boost was scheduled to begin in May 2010. Fifteen new sites were to be chosen to begin the program in October, in addition to the 20 in California. Applicants are required to complete an online needs/resource assessment and to submit a letter of support from a senior administrator (for example, the chief medical officer or chief nursing officer). For more information on Project BOOST, go online to http://www.hospitalmedicine.org/BOOST or e-mail BOOST@hospitalmedicine.org.

CASE STUDY: ONCOLOGY CARE AT THE INTERFACE BETWEEN HOSPITAL AND COMMUNITY CARE IN ISRAEL

Patients with chronic conditions and complex care needs often experience breakdowns in care when making transitions across care settings. Studies from various countries show that cancer patients are no exception and that breakdowns occur across the cancer care trajectory.[8–10] Research also shows that there is uncertainty about the division of responsibility for the various aspects of patient care between primary care physicians and oncologists, as well as differing professional strategies in cancer management.[11]

According to Efrat Shadmi, Ph.D., R.N., from the Cheryl Spencer Department of Nursing, Faculty of Social Welfare and Health Sciences at Haifa University, Israel, these research findings have been supported by anecdotal patient reports on their perilous journeys through the health care system. "In many cases, patients report not knowing who to turn to with questions or concerns, and feeling frustration about omissions or duplications in their care," Shadmi says.[12]

"In Israel, like in many other countries, cancer patients receive their care from several types of providers, including hospital and community-based specialists and primary care providers," says Shadmi. "By law, all Israelis are covered by universal health insurance and belong to one of four Health Funds where they receive most of their care, with the exception of hospitalizations in government or publicly owned hospitals."[12] Previous Israeli research shows that patients discharged from general medical units experienced breakdowns in care when transitioning from the hospital to community care.[13]

Shadmi and Drs. Hanna Admi, Lea Ungar, Nurit Naveh, and Michael Kaffman, along with Ms. Ella Muller and professor Shmuel Reis, undertook a multimethod approach to studying the quality of oncology care at the interface between care at a large tertiary facility in the northern part of Israel (which serves a large heterogeneous catchment of two million people) and community primary care.[14] The study was conducted during the years 2007–2008 and was funded by the Israel National Institute for Healthcare Policy. The study had three purposes[14]:

1. To increase awareness of the various barriers that oncology patients face when making transitions across care settings
2. To evaluate the different approaches of hospital and community care providers
3. To specifically assess whether special population groups, such as minority ethnic patients and new immigrants, face additional challenges

The Israeli oncology study included qualitative interviews with patients and their caregivers, primary care physicians, oncologists, nurses at the hospital and at primary care clinics, social workers, and health administrators. Study questionnaires were completed by 422 patients who had been recently discharged from the hospital.

Results

Findings from the study offer a comprehensive picture of the consequences of dealing with a complex and fragmented health care system from the point of view of both oncology patients and health personnel. "The study indicates the importance of the role of the family physician in continuity of care," says Shadmi. "Performance of coordination activities by primary care physicians was suboptimal, with integration aspects of care being rated amongst the lowest of six common primary care attributes, including integration, access to care, whole person knowledge, interpersonal care, trust in physician, [and] communication."[12]

Patients' average rating of the quality of transition from the hospital to the community was 76 on the Care Transitions Measure™ scale, which ranges from 0 to 100 (*see* Chapter 6 for more information about the Care Transitions Measure). "Primary care physician involvement was found to be the most significant variable affecting the evaluation of the transition from the hospital to the community," Shadmi says. "In cases where physicians discussed the discharge recommendations with their patients, the understanding of treatment aspects related to the hospital–community interface was better."[12]

With regard to the special populations included in this study, new immigrants from Russia and other parts of the former Soviet Union rated their physicians lowest on all primary care domains, as compared with the general nonimmigrant population. However, according to patient reports, primary care physicians who treated Russian-speaking patients were more likely to discuss discharge recommendations with their patients than were physicians who treated Hebrew-speaking patients. "This is an encouraging example of the practice of culturally tailored care, indicating that primary care physicians were putting in extra effort to making sure their non-native Hebrew-speaking patients understood the discharge instructions," says Shadmi.[12]

Discussion

According to Shadmi, the Israeli oncology study has not yet resulted in specific policy changes. However, an important change was initiated by the largest health fund in Israel—the insurer and provider of more than 60% of the study's participants. Toward the end of the study period, but unrelated to the study itself, the health fund canceled requirements for special preauthorizations for various oncology procedures, including emergency department visits and hospitalizations. "This change had an important positive effect on both patients and providers who were burdened with the need to deal with the complex bureaucracy involved with preauthorization requirements," Shadmi says.[12]

The findings of this study suggest several policy implications regarding care of oncology patients during the transition between the hospital and the community. First, given the significant positive correlation found between the discussion of the discharge recommendations with the primary care physician and the patient's understanding of treatment goals, the visit to the patient's primary care physician should be viewed as an opportunity to evaluate the patient's level of understanding of the recommendations and the degree of compatibility of those recommendations to the rest of the treatment, and as an opportunity to make sure that the treatment program is clear to both the patient and the primary care physician.

Second, examining the differences between various groups of the population, it is clear that the group reporting the most difficulties consists of immigrants who are coping with communication difficulties and culturally unsuitable treatment.

In light of these findings, it is important to examine the objective difficulties that immigrants face, in addition to dealing with cancer, and the unique needs of this population in order develop appropriate interventions—for example, patient navigation programs—that are already being used in many countries around the world.

CASE STUDY:
U.S. VETERANS AFFAIRS
SHIFT HANDOFF TOOL

In the spring of 2006, Divya Shroff, M.D., associate chief of staff, Informatics, at the U.S. Veterans Affairs (VA) Medical Center in Washington, DC, realized that handoffs (transitions of care) at the medical center were not being done as well as they could be. "At the time I was an academic hospitalist," Shroff says. "When I was rounding with the covering team on the weekend, I might hear someone say something like, 'Mr. Jones is on antibiotic treatment day four,' when I knew that wasn't right. There were a lot of discrepancies in the way handoffs were being done. Some people were using Excel [spread]sheets, some were using e-mail. People were often cutting and pasting from the EMR [electronic medical record, also called electronic health record]. It was pretty hodgepodge."[15]

Knowing that its system had flaws and that The Joint Commission was preparing to release a National Patient Safety Goal that would require standardized handoff processes for transitions of care, the VA's National Center for Patient Safety began to look at physician-to-physician transitions. Noel Eldridge, a team leader at the national center, put out a query to all the VA centers asking if anyone had a standardized process and found that the Indianapolis VA had a system being used that pulled information from the VA's electronic health record, the Computerized Patient Record System (CPRS).

Developing the Handoff Tool

The VA's National Center for Patient Safety put together a six-site collaborative to address the issue. Programmers from Indianapolis were included in the collaborative. "We started with the form from Indianapolis," Shroff says. "We went ahead and tested it out in [Washington,] D.C. as the test site, and the house staff revolted. The form wasn't exactly what they wanted. The patient information was in paragraph form, so it wasn't very user-friendly. The information was there, but you sometimes had to go through several pages to find what you were looking for."[15]

In the fall of 2006, the collaborative put together a team of programmers and clinicians. "We began looking at how other academic programs were doing handoffs," says Shroff. "We

found one standardized system for a non-EMR-based health care system that was developed by a resident named Daniel Rosenthal at George Washington University and was in popular use by the house staff there. We knew we could use that as a basic template. We just needed to take that concept and make it VA-friendly. We needed to look at what should be standardized and what could be pulled from CPRS."[15] The team developed a list of key elements to become a part of the final product, including the following[15]:

- Team identifiers
- Appropriate patient identifiers
- Patient presentation
- Active problem and medication list
- Allergies
- Code status
- Potential problems that may arise over the next 18 to 24 hours
- What to do when problems arise

How the Tool Works

When someone clicks on the handoff tool, an automated list of patients pops up on the screen. Alternately, the provider can create his or her own list of patients. When the provider clicks on the name of a patient, a working page pops up (*see* Figure 7-5, page 137). After the information is complete, a printout can be generated to use during the transition of care (*see* Figure 7-6, page 138).

Implementation

In the spring of 2007, the Shift Handoff Tool went live at the Veterans Affairs Medical Center in Washington, DC. "We first implemented it on our medicine floors," Shroff says. "Then we tweaked it some and rolled it out to the rest of the testing sites." Following implementation, the team presented its findings at a national VA conference. "The tool created a lot of buzz," says Shroff. "The VA decided to make it a national tool. It was released nationally in 2008."[15]

According to Shroff, one of the biggest challenges to implementation was trying to convince physicians to continue to test something that had not worked in the past. "We tested so many versions," Shroff says, "especially in [Washington] D.C. We had to work hard to keep everyone inspired and to make sure they could see the final vision. Having the same hospitalist team members every week really helped."[15]

Another challenge the VA faced when implementing the Shift Handoff Tool was explaining to programmers why things

Figure 7-5. Handoff Tool Patient Screen

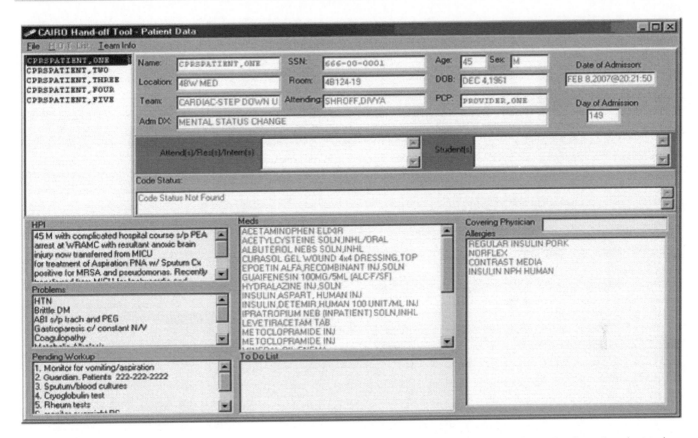

When a provider is working within the electronic health record, a screen is autopopulated with information from the electronic health record, with spaces for free-text input to help with information on the transition of care.

Source: Veterans Affairs Medical Center, Washington, DC. Used with permission.

needed to be changed. "Initially, the programmers didn't understand why people didn't like what was being used in Indianapolis," Shroff says. "Programmers don't always come from clinical backgrounds, so we had to let them know how doctors think and work. We had to make sure we were coming across as giving them constructive feedback rather than attacking them while developing a standardized solution."[15]

Results

The Veterans Administration evaluated its Shift Handoff Tool by pre- and postimplementation surveys at VA Medical Centers in Washington, DC, and Iowa City, Iowa, in an effort led by Dr. Jaclyn Anderson at Iowa City. "We collected what people were using as handoff tools before we implemented the program, then asked them questions about how they felt about the type and quality of information they were receiving during handoff and the amount of time it would take," says Shroff. "We surveyed them again after the tool was implemented. Satisfaction had greatly increased."[15]

In August 2008, the Veterans Affairs Medical Center in Washington, DC, received a 2009 Most Wired innovator award from *Hospitals & Health Networks* magazine, a publication of the American Hospital Association, for its Shift Handoff Tool.

Figure 7-6. Handoff Tool

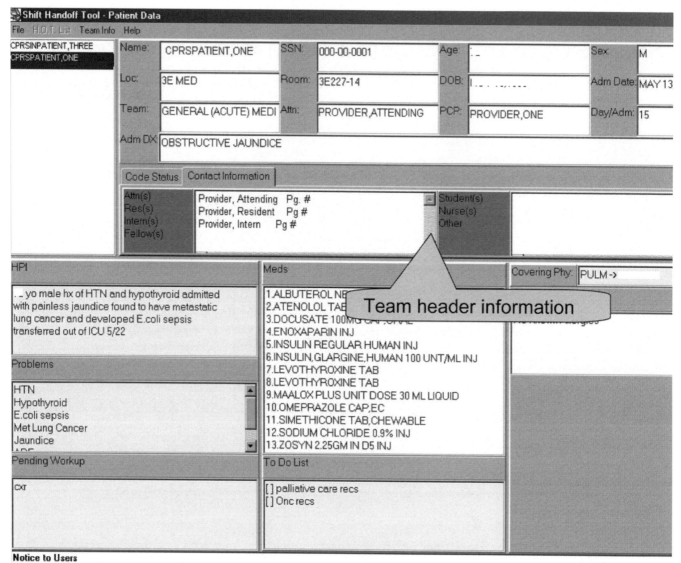

When patient information is complete, a printout from the handoff tool can be generated to help with transitions of care.

Source: Veterans Affairs Medical Center, Washington, D.C. Used with permission.

CASE STUDY: PUTNAM HOSPITAL CENTER'S ANTICOAGULANT THERAPY PROGRAM

Due to the complexity of dosing and monitoring of anticoagulants, anticoagulant therapy is a high-risk treatment that commonly leads to adverse drug events. In 2007, Putnam Hospital Center, an acute care hospital in Carmel, New York, began an initiative to improve the safety of anticoagulant therapy. As part of its initiative, the hospital implemented a pharmacist-driven approach to managing warfarin orders.[16]

Putnam Hospital Center's revised warfarin management process focused on three areas[16]:
1. Ensuring a baseline International Normalized Ratio (INR) for every warfarin patient
2. Improving communication between the physician, pharmacist, nurse, and dietitian regarding patients using warfarin
3. Creating a system to facilitate daily monitoring of INR by the pharmacist

Ensuring a Baseline INR

When warfarin is prescribed for a patient at Putnam Hospital Center, the order is electronically scanned and transmitted to the pharmacy. The pharmacist reviews the order and checks for a baseline INR. If there is no baseline INR in the patient's record, the prescriber has 24 hours to order one. If the order is not received within 24 hours, the pharmacist calls the prescriber to remind him or her to order an INR. The pharmacist also documents whether or not a baseline INR was ordered, which allows the hospital to measure whether baseline INRs are being ordered in a timely manner.

Improving Communication Between Providers

When the pharmacist enters a warfarin order into Putnam Hospital Center's computer system, he or she also enters a "marker" for warfarin, which shows up on the paper-based medication administration record (MAR).[16] The marker serves as a reminder to the nurse and other providers to continue to monitor the INR and to periodically check for new warfarin orders and INR results for the patient. The marker allows for continuous communication during the patient's hospital visit because the pharmacist can quickly communicate information to other providers without having to contact them directly. The marker also assists providers with discharge planning because all care providers have quick access to the patient's status, INR level, and current anticoagulant dose.

Daily INR Monitoring

Putnam Hospital Center created a process to remind pharmacists to monitor INRs on a daily basis. The reminder comes through the pharmacist's automated daily work queue. If a patient's INR value is greater than 3, the pharmacist calls the prescriber for new orders. New orders may include a dose reduction, discontinuation of therapy, or an alternative therapy. The pharmacist then enters the new order and updates the marker to communicate the change to the patient's other providers.

Evaluation

By the end of 2008, on average, 96% of patients receiving warfarin had a baseline INR within 24 hours of therapy initiation.[16] Although no formal surveys have yet been conducted to determine whether communication between nurses and pharmacists has improved as a result of this initiative, informal staff feedback suggests that it has.

CASE STUDY: IMPROVING COMMUNICATION BETWEEN HOME HEALTH AGENCIES AND HEALTH PLANS

In March 1996, senior leaders and case managers from the Home Health Care Association of Massachusetts (now the Home Care Alliance of Massachusetts [HCAM]) and the Massachusetts Association of Health Plans (MAHP) held a meeting to discuss how they could better work together for the good of their patients. "At that time, Massachusetts had a higher percentage of managed care organizations than other parts of the country," says Helen Siegel, R.N., M.S., M.B.A., director of regulatory and clinical affairs, HCAM. "There was a lot of tension between the home health agencies who were used to doing their own case management and the case managers at the health plans who were now telling them how to manage their patients. It was a difficult situation. Both sides decided it was time to start a dialogue to see what we could do to make things better."[17]

According to Mary Ann Preskul-Ricca, M.P.P., public affairs coordinator, MAHP, prior to the meeting, communication between the two groups was very strained. "When the home health agencies were requesting authorizations, there was not a lot of open communication," she says. "The meeting was a safe place for both sides to get together and have a frank discussion about how we could improve communication."[17]

The year after the meeting, the two groups got together again for a panel discussion. Following that meeting, communication began to improve, and so the two groups decided to form the Health Plan/Home Health Partnership to continue their dialogue on an ongoing basis. "Once the home health case managers realized that both entities would be managing the patients together, things began to improve," says Siegel. "Both groups began to realize that part of the problem was different forms and authorization processes. So a subgroup of the partnership sat down and wrote a universal form [*see* Figure 7-7, pages 141–142]. They did it in about an hour, and everyone on both sides thought it was great."[17]

After the form was developed, the partnership held a training session for all health plan case managers and home health case managers. "At the meeting, we explained in detail what was on the form and why," Preskul-Ricca says. "Understanding why a particular question is being asked has helped with compliance."[17]

Results

The partnership continues to meet on a quarterly basis and holds an annual forum that is open to a wider audience of health plan and home health staff. "Every year we have a 'Connect the Dots' program on a topic that's appropriate for both groups," says Siegel. "Now that we're at the point where people are working well together, the focus has shifted from how we can better communicate with each other to what we can do for our patients."[17]

Preskul-Ricca adds, "The topic ideas come from the partnership members. They know what's going on in the field and what we need to focus on."[17] Some topics discussed at previous meetings include the expedited appeal process for Medicare Advantage, the Medicare Notice of Non-Coverage, and motivational interviewing techniques to achieve patient adherence.

According to Siegel, both groups have undergone a transformation since the partnership began. "There's a lot more trust," she says. "When the universal form was first developed, the health plans were monitoring things very closely. Now that we're all working together, there's more trust on both sides. The home health agencies have learned a lot from the health plans and they've gotten better about managing patient care, so the health plans are allowing them to develop their own care plans. Because the health plans have seen that the home health agencies are providing good patient care and that patients are having good outcomes, there's not as much micromanaging."[17]

Preskul-Ricca offers the following advice to others who want to improve relationships either within their own organization or between organizations that are working together toward similar goals. "Get everyone in the room and start talking," she says. "It always goes back to communication. As long as you have a group that's committed to working things out and providing good patient care, you'll be successful."[17]

Figure 7-7. Universal Health Plan/Home Health Authorization Form

UNIVERSAL HEALTH PLAN/ HOME HEALTH AUTHORIZATION FORM

S.OC. Date: ___/___/___ **Initial:** ☐ **Reauthorization:**___/___/___
Agency D/C Date:___/___/___ : Anticipated ☐ Actual ☐ MD Agrees: Y/N Patient Agrees: Y/N

Patient Information
Name:_____
S.O.C. Address:_____
_____
Telephone #:_____
DOB:___/___/___
Homebound: Y/N Why?_____
Diagnosis:_____
Surgery: N/A_____
Patient Prognosis:
Poor / Guarded / Fair / Good / Very Good /
Excellent / <6 months to live / Terminal.
MD Information
Ordering MD:_____
MD Phone#:_____
PCP:_____
Date of Next MD Visit:___/___/___
Health Plan Information
Health Plan Name:_____
Insurance #:_____
Health Plan CM:_____
Initial Auth#:_____
Telephone #:_____ Fax #:_____

Agency Information
Agency Name:_____
Provider Number:_____
Contact:_____
Telephone #:_____ Fax#:_____
DME/Supplies/IV/Lab
Vendor Name:_____
Community Resources_____
_____
Caregiver Information
Name:_____
Relationship:_____
Type of Assistance:_____
Teachable/Not Teachable:_____
Primary Phone#:_____

Maternity Care N/A ☐
Delivery Date___/___/___Time Of Delivery__:__
Discharge Date___/___/___Time of Discharge__:__

Current Functional Status

Cognitive	Dress Lower Extremities	Bathing	Toileting	Ambulation
☐Alert/Oriented	☐ Independent	☐ Independent	☐ Independent	☐ Independent
☐ Impaired	☐ Requires assist	☐ Requires assist	☐ Requires assist	☐ Requires assist
☐ Disoriented	☐ Unable	☐ Unable	☐ Unable	☐ Unable

Service Request	From	To	# Of Visits	Frequency	Auth # Visits	Health Plan Auth #
RN						
HHA/Hrs&Visits						
PT						
OT						
ST						
MSW						
Other						

Communication

Comments:_____
_____
_____
_____
_____

Name:_____ **Title:**_____ **Date:** ___/___/___

Developed by Health Plan/Home Health Partnership of Massachusetts. © Do not reproduce without permission of the Partnership **Mar 1,2006.**

(continued on page 142)

Figure 7-7. Universal Health Plan/Home Health Authorization Form, *continued*

Page 2   *Patient Name:*_____*Agency:*_____*Auth #*_____

SKILLED NURSING D/C Date:___/___/___ Anticipated ☐ Actual ☐
*Clinical summary:*_____
_____
_____
_____
_____

Reason for Home Health Aide Services:_____
_____

Wound Care N/A☐	Wound 1	Wound 2	Wound 3
Location			
Appearance			
Measurement			
Drainage			
TX and Frequency			

Medications: Compliant: Y/N   Teachable Patient: Y/N   Med List Attached: NA/Y
Goals/Plan for this Authorization Period: _____
_____
_____

Barriers to Achieve Goals/Plan: _____
_____

Interventions: _____
_____
_____

Signature:_____ **Title:**_____ **Department:**_____ **Date:**___/___/___

OTHER SKILLED DISCIPLINES D/C Date: ___/___/___ Anticipated ☐ Actual ☐
Please complete a separate pg. 2 when more than one skilled discipline providing care
PT _____ **OT**_____ **ST**_____ **MSW** _____**Other**_____
Reason for Home Health Aide Services:_____

*Clinical summary?*_____
_____

Goals/Plan for this authorization period:_____
_____
_____

Barriers to achieve goals/plan: _____

Interventions: _____
_____
_____

Signature: _____ **Title:**_____ **Department:**_____ **Date:**___/___/___

Source: Home Care Alliance of Massachusetts/Massachusetts Association of Health Plans. Used with permission.

Case Study: University of California San Francisco's Home Health Care Referral Process

The home health care referral process at the University of California San Francisco (UCSF) began in 1998 as an educational tool for staff working in the medical center. "At the time, there was a need identified to reach out and provide more information to case managers and physicians as to what services a skilled home health care agency could provide for patients," says Joan Spicer, R.N., Ph.D., director, UCSF Medical Center Case Management/Social Work/Home Health Care. "We were concerned that some referrals were not appropriate and that perhaps other patients who might benefit from home health care services were not being referred, so we developed a 'standard order set' that would help to educate prescribers as to what options are available when referring patients for home health care."[18] (*See* Figure 7-8, pages 144–145).

When the interdisciplinary team at UCSF identifies a patient who may benefit from home health care services, the patient's options of agencies are then reviewed with the patient based on the patient's payer source. The patient then makes a choice as to which home health care agency he or she would prefer to use. "After the patient makes a choice, the case manager works with the physician to obtain orders using the standard order set," says Spicer. "At the same time, the case manager also makes contact with the home health agency to do an initial review of the patient's medical history, diagnoses, and home care needs. For home health agencies in our area, the medical center is able to communicate patient information electronically. If the patient's choice is to use the UCSF home health care agency, the agency has access to the patient's EMR [electronic medical record]."[18]

Staff Education

After the standard order set was developed, both case managers and providers were educated about how to use the form. "At UCSF Medical Center, the case managers are the primary liaisons to the providers, so they worked to educate providers based on each individual patient's needs," Spicer says.[18]

Since the standard order set was implemented, it has twice been revised. "The first revision incorporated orders for skilled nursing facilities and transfer patients," says Spicer. "The most recent revision was done as part of UCSF's participation in the Society of Hospital Medicine's Project BOOST program, with UCSF physicians, case managers, home care nurses, and physical therapists collaborating on the revisions."[18]

Results

The form is now used for all referrals from UCSF Medical Center to home health care agencies. "The standardized order set has made it more efficient for the UCSF Home Health Care intake nurse to ensure that the referral and the orders are appropriate and specific to the patient's clinical needs and to the criteria for home health care services," Spicer says.[18]

Figure 7-8. UCSF Discharge Orders for All Home Care, Skilled Nursing Facility, and Transfer Patients

UCSF Medical Center

UNIT NUMBER

PT. NAME

BIRTHDATE

DISCHARGE ORDERS FOR ALL HOME CARE, SNF, AND TRANSFER PATIENTS

Complete Pages 1 and 2 for
ALL Home Care, SNF, and Transfer Patients

LOCATION   DATE

Home Health and Skilled Nursing Facility Orders

☐ Home Health   OR   ☐ SNF Transfer

☐ **A nurse is needed for the following services**	☐ **Wound Care:** *Please Describe location of wound and basics of wound care.*

☐ **TPN, or Enteric Feeds:** *Please provide details, nutrition type, and route. A prescription must be included with any order for TPN or enteric feeds.*

☐ Include order for Line Care. Line Type/Location: _____ .
☐ Include order for Tube Care. Tube Type/Location: _____ .

☐ **IV medications:** *List Medications with Dose, Frequency, Start Date (post-d/c), End Date. A prescription must be included with this order.*

Drug:	Dose:	freq.	Date Range:
Drug:	Dose:	freq.	Date Range:
Drug:	Dose:	freq.	Date Range:

☐ Include order for Line Care. Line Type/Location: _____ .

☐ **Patient Assessment, Intervention, and Education by an RN (for Home Care only):** *Please describe nature of assessment or education that requires an RN.*

☐ **Physical Therapy**	☐ **Patient Goals:** *Please describe briefly & specify any mobility restrictions*
☐ **Speech Therapy**	☐ **Patient Goals:** *Please describe briefly.*

If you are requesting one of the needs above, your patient is also eligible for:

☐ Medical Social Worker: Assessment, intervention related to social and emotional function & referral to community services
☐ Home Safety Evaluation
☐ Occupational Therapy
☐ Laboratory tests to be reported to the Responsible Physician: *Please describe Test, Initial Date and Frequency*

Test	Start Date	Freq.
Test	Start Date	Freq.
Test	Start Date	Freq.

Additional Discharge Instructions for Service Providers:
May include nursing orders for Home Health/SNF. Do not use this area for meds or patient instructions.

YELLOW - NURSING COPY   ORIGINAL - MEDICAL RECORD COPY

105-0277 (Rev. 04/10) WorkflowOne

DISCHARGE ORDERS FOR ALL HOME CARE, SNF, AND TRANSFER PATIENTS Page 1 of 2

Figure 7-8. UCSF Discharge Orders for All Home Care, Skilled Nursing Facility, and Transfer Patients, *continued*

UC_SF Medical Center

UNIT NUMBER	
PT. NAME	
BIRTHDATE	
LOCATION	DATE

DISCHARGE ORDERS FOR ALL HOME CARE, SNF, AND TRANSFER PATIENTS
Complete Pages 1 and 2 for
ALL Home Care, SNF, and Transfer Patients

Responsible Physician: will be responsible for Home Care orders and receiving patient condition follow up.
For residents or NPs you must put the supervising clinic attending or MD.

Attending Name:	License:
Resident/NP Name:	UPIN:
Phone:	Fax:	Pager:

NOTE: You must contact the physician above prior to listing them as the responsible MD.

☐ *I have contacted the Attending above who agrees to accept home care orders. Date:*

Durable Medical Equipment Orders

Assistive Equipment	☐ Wheelchair ☐ 3-in-1 Commode ☐ Hospital Bed ☐ 3-Wheel Walker
	☐ Pressure Relieving Mattress ☐ Continuous Passive Motion Machine
Respiratory Care	☐ Oxygen _____ L/min ☐ Concentrator ☐ Humidifier ☐ Nebulizer
	☐ Portable Suction ☐ CPAP/BiPAP, settings: _____
	☐ **Room Air Saturation** _____ *(Required for Medicare patients <88%)*
	☐ **ABG results** _____ *(Required for Medical patients PO$_2$ <55)*

Additional Discharge Orders for Home Care or Transfer

Weight Bearing Status	☐ LEFT or RIGHT *(circle one)* ☐ UPPER or LOWER extremity *(circle one)*
	☐ Full ☐ Partial _____ % ☐ Non-weight bearing
Pain Management	☐ Assess pain frequently ☐ Use relaxation techniques
	☐ See Discharge prescription ☐ Other
Glucose Monitoring	☐ Before Meals and at Bedtime
	☐ Other: _____
GU/Bowel Care	☐ Foley ☐ Stoma bag ☐ Straight cath every 8hrs ☐ Ostomy bag
	☐ Other GU/Bowel Care: _____
Respiratory Care	☐ Tracheostomy: Size: _____ Date Placed: _____
Orthotics or Splint	☐ TLSO ☐ Cybertec 1000 ☐ Multipodus Boot ☐ AFO ☐ Upper Extremity Splint
	☐ Other Type of Brace: _____
	☐ Brace at all times ☐ Brace removed for showering ☐ Brace when out of bed
	☐ Other: _____
Precautions	☐ Skin Breakdown ☐ Log Roll every _____ hrs ☐ Falls ☐ Aspiration
	☐ Infection/Organism: _____

Prescribing Physician Information

PRESCRIBER'S NAME:		PAGER:	CO-SIGNER'S NAME:		PAGER:
PRESCRIBER'S SIGNATURE:			CO-SIGNER'S SIGNATURE:		
CA LIC#:	DEA#:	DATE:	CA LIC#:	DEA#:	DATE:

105-0277 (Rev. 04/10) WorkflowOne   ORIGINAL - MEDICAL RECORD COPY   YELLOW - NURSING COPY

DISCHARGE ORDERS FOR ALL HOME CARE, SNF, AND TRANSFER PATIENTS Page 2 of 2

This form helps ensure that referrals to home health care agencies are appropriate. It also serves as prescriber orders.

Source: University of California San Francisco Medical Center. Used with permission.

CASE STUDY: DEVELOPING AND EVALUATING A CLASSROOM-BASED INTERVENTION TO IMPROVE COMMUNICATION AMONG STAFF MEMBERS IN A DANISH HOSPITAL

In May 2006, a study was initiated in a Danish hospital to determine whether there was a need for a curriculum to improve hospital staff communication and patient safety, and if so, what the characteristics of that curriculum should be. The preparatory phase in the clinical departments began in June 2007.

The study was initiated based on the following factors:

- Recommendations from the landmark study *To Err Is Human: Building a Safer Health System*[19] about improving teamwork in health care and establishing interdisciplinary team-training programs for providers in order to strengthen patient safety
- Endorsement of the recommendations in *To Err Is Human* by leading international health care organizations[20–22]
- A Danish adverse event study[23] that revealed that the patient safety problem in Denmark, as well as internationally, is equivalent to that of the United States

Denmark currently has an 85% publicly financed health care sector. Danish hospital physicians are employed by the hospital and affiliated with certain departments and floors, rather than having private clinics in the community and tending to their own patients in different hospitals.[24,25] Nurses routinely make rounds with physicians. Salaries are relatively uniform among staff of the same discipline. However, the medical department leader and other experienced physicians earn approximately twice as much as nurses with the same experience. Continuity of care within hospitals is the responsibility of the organization.

"In the American health care system, patients select their own physicians who run their own businesses and admit patients to their hospital of choice," says Louise Rabøl, M.D., Copenhagen.[26] "Physicians often care for their own inpatients and frequently round without nurses. Some subspecialists

earn a salary that is 10 times higher than that of a resident and 15 times higher than that of a nurse."[26]

"These structural and cultural differences can impact communication and teamwork," says Rabøl. "For example, there are differences in how authorities are approached, how actions of team leaders are questioned, and how new inventions like checklists and communication structuring are readily accepted by the learners."[26]

A needs assessment was conducted between May 2006 and September 2007 to determine the needs and potential structure of a Danish curriculum. The needs assessment consisted of the following three elements:

1. An analysis of the most severe patient safety incidents in Copenhagen hospitals from 2004 to 2006
2. Four multidisciplinary focus group interviews with staff
3. A systematic literature review of the results of multi-disciplinary classroom-based team-training interventions for hospital staff

"Allowing for both hindsight and confirmation bias, the analysis of severe patient safety incidents concluded that erroneous verbal communication between staff members was either a root cause or a contributing factor in more than half of the incidents," says Rabøl. "Loss of information during transitions of care, particularly during patient transfers, was described as the most frequent characteristic of the incidents. This was described as being caused by lack of structuring and proceduralizing transitions of care, particularly during the patient transfer process and during transitions conducted by telephone."[26]

Analysis of the focus group interviews uncovered that staff members considered awaiting and combining information from two chart systems, handing over information, and getting sufficient information when calling someone to be the main challenges to communication because lack of information and misunderstandings often led to delays and sometimes to errors. "The main promoters of safe verbal communication were established frameworks for communication, mutual knowledge, a culture that allows all staff members to speak up, experience in getting the message through, and focus on teamwork and communication," says Rabøl. "The main barriers were lack of standard assignments, different agendas for the patient among staff groups, and communication challenges due to interruptions and multitasking."[26]

The systematic literature review showed that classroom-based team-training interventions yielded positive results on participant reaction, learning, and behavior. "The results at the clinical level are still very limited," Rabøl says. "However, many of the study designs were weak, and few interventions were evaluated after the training itself."[26]

During the needs assessment process, a hospitalwide patient safety cultural survey (conducted without relation to the study itself) revealed an overall high degree of trust, support, and openness among staff. Only a small percentage of staff members said they did not speak up when they had concerns about safety. However, almost 25% said that information had been lost during shift change, and more than half reported that information was lost when patients were being transferred between units.[27] This finding was confirmed by reports from the departments to the Danish national incident reporting system.[28]

The needs assessment was followed by establishment of a draft curriculum that underwent three cycles of systematic curriculum planning, pilot testing, analysis, and revision. The pilot tests made clear that there was a need for customization and that all staff groups and specialties had a need for training. The pilot tests also stressed the importance of the following:

- Structuring and standardizing communication
- Teamwork at the expense of assertion tools (tools that legitimize speaking up to authorities if there is a safety concern)
- The need for thorough adaptation of cases, photos, and videos—which were originally in English, from American settings, and included a mix of surgical and medical cases—to local conditions and participating staff groups
- Introduction of tools and strategies at the organizational level instead of at the department level because patients often cross unit borders
- Follow-up
- Role playing and feedback
- The use of participant experience, small group discussions, humor, videos, and short breaks to increase attention and reduce resistance

Implementation

Following the needs assessment, a multidisciplinary curriculum was developed for hospital staff. The curriculum consisted of the following five learning modules:

1. *Introduction to Patient Safety:* This module introduced staff to basic patient safety data and to a "systems approach" to improving safety, as opposed to blaming individuals for errors.
2. *The Human Factor:* This module used examples to help staff see that although all human beings make mistakes, a team approach can improve safety.
3. *Communication:* This module presented frameworks and checklists for safer verbal communication and allowed staff members to practice using these and to receive feedback on their performance.
4. *Teamwork:* This module outlined the roles of the team leader and team members. In a nonclinical challenge, teams were given the opportunity to use the tools and strategies.
5. *Implementation and Evaluation:* This module introduced the plan for implementation. Staff members were given the opportunity to make suggestions and provide feedback.

"The curriculum was established as both a two-day train-the-trainer program and a conventional one-day program to meet the needs for local adaptation and ownership," says Rabøl.[26]

To increase the likelihood of transfer of communications during transitions of care, staff members were provided with a pocket-size handbook[29] that included the following checklists:

- **Improvement in handover:** The purpose of this checklist is to raise awareness of the importance of reliable information exchange, to give staff members a visual reminder of important information to be transferred during transitions of care, to help staff members provide an analysis of the patient's condition and to clarify patient needs during transitions of care, and to provide a standardized method of communication to the receiving party.
- **Improvement in transfer of patients:** This checklist is a more detailed version of the improvement in handover checklist. It provides all the above, plus information about the patient's medications, special safety issues related to transfer, tests or procedures that are pending, who is escorting the patient, informed consent, and who is responsible for which aspects of the patient's care during transfer.
- **Improvement in teamwork:** The purpose of this checklist is to raise awareness about the roles of all team members and the importance of reliable information exchange, to give staff members a visual reminder of important information to be transferred during transitions of care, to make sure that all team members understand what the others are doing and why, and to make sure that team members speak up if a safety issue is identified.

The complete version of the curriculum was tested in a controlled intervention among staff members in a department for cardiology and pulmonary diseases at a university hospital in the Capital Region of Denmark in 2007. The unit had 151 staff members who were involved in exchanging patient data. Participation was mandatory. Training took place during four eight-hour seminars.

"The follow-up campaign started immediately after the first session and lasted until April 2008, a period of seven months," Rabøl says. "During the follow-up campaign, supporting materials were evaluated and replaced when needed. The local project group, rather than the frontline staff, received coaching. This setup was chosen to encourage local engagement and to simulate a realistic implementation at a public hospital, where full-time coaching by an outsider is not feasible."[26]

Implementation Challenges

Rabøl admits that there were some challenges to implementing the new curriculum. "Senior leadership and midlevel manager backup was not very visible, and this limited implementation," she says. "Overall, the effect of training also began to fade after an initial phase of high enthusiasm. Both staff and leaders described that there was a lack of follow-up and local ownership."[26] To help overcome these challenges, staff requested the following:

- Forcing functions (for example, a field on the anaesthesiologists' report that indicates that a briefing has been completed in order for the procedure to continue)
- Refresher courses
- Training of new staff
- Structural changes (for example, more time between shifts to give nurses sufficient time for a proper transition at shift change)
- Training of staff in other departments
- A project group (to allow for multidisciplinary involvement and thereby a higher degree of ownership)
- Inclusion of communicative issues in clinical discussions
- Organizational guidelines to underscore the importance of the tools and strategies

Use of the curriculum was also inhibited by the pressure of other tasks, such as an organizationwide accreditation survey and simultaneous implementation of other new initiatives, and by the difficulty of breaking old habits. More-experienced staff believed that the intervention was useful for others but unnecessary for themselves. These issues, as well as staff requests, will be addressed during the next phase of implementation. "My intervention became a forerunner of hospitalwide implementation," says Rabøl. "At the hospital level, they have used the train-the-trainer approach. This approach has allowed for a high degree of customization. This intervention is ongoing, and the results of this evaluation will be used in yet another round of intervention that will take place in the fall [of] 2010."[26]

Evaluation

This curriculum was evaluated at the following levels:
- The participants' reactions to training
- Participant knowledge immediately after training
- Participant knowledge two to four months after training
- Participants' self-rating of their own use of tools and strategies
- Participants' rating of their peers' use of tools and strategies
- A controlled observation of communication after the intervention
- A controlled study of the level of patient safety incidents six months before and six months after the study

One month after the intervention, staff members expressed a belief that training had strengthened patient safety, teamwork, communication, assertion, listening skills, and patient transfer safety. They also believed that the intervention had leadership support. A controlled postintervention observation study showed a significantly higher quality of communication among caregivers. However, the results were limited to only a few individuals. A controlled, structured before-and-after record audit of patient safety initiatives did not show positive clinical results. In semistructured interviews, staff endorsed the concept but criticized the lack of follow-up. This criticism is being addressed during the hospitalwide intervention. The hospital continues to explore its use of the curriculum.

Case Study: Transition from the Hospital to Home Health Services in Qatar

When patients are ready to be discharged from the hospital but still require health care services in the home, it is important to make the transition of care from hospital to home as smooth as possible for patients and family members. At the Hamad Medical Corporation (HMC), in Doha, Qatar, staff members from the hospital and home health services have been taking steps to ensure that patients and families receive timely, appropriate, and safe care in the home immediately after discharge.

HMC is comprised of five hospitals and also provides many other services, such as home health care. In Qatar, health care is primarily funded by the government, and the HMC is a government entity that is overseen by the Supreme Council of Health.[30] Home health services is a relatively new service offered by HMC, says Vicki Alexandra Scruby, assistant executive director, Home Health Services at HMC. "In the past there was some care provision in patients' homes, but the service was somewhat fragmented without an explicit structure," says Scruby. "Now, our services are more comprehensive and structured with case management, and we've expanded to serve more patients. Patients and families are very receptive to the service. They like the concept of receiving care in the home."[31]

Note: *All five HMC hospitals have been accredited by Joint Commission International (JCI). Home Health Services was accredited by JCI's Care Continuum program—designed to assess a variety of community-based care settings such as home care, assisted living, long term care, and hospice care—on 28 October 2009.*

Implementation

To improve the transition of care from the hospital to the home, staff reviewed case management and discharge planning processes. "We introduced a liaison case manager position within the hospital to facilitate transitions from the hospital to the community with home health services," says Scruby. "New referrals to home health services come to the liaison's attention before patients are discharged. The liaison

identifies the high-risk patients and will assess those patients and family members before discharge in order to proactively plan for the patients' care in the home."[31] The liaison will assess the patient's needs for medical equipment and devices, wound care treatments, venipuncture and intravenous medications, mechanical ventilation, and so on. If necessary, a home visit to assess the environment may be initiated as well.

Many patients continue to receive home health services for several months or years, and these patients may return to the hospital for care at certain times. "Every day, we receive the admission list from the emergency department so that we can identify any of our patients and get involved in their discharge process as well," says Scruby. "For our existing patients and new referrals, it is important to be proactive in planning care for patients in the home. In this way, we can prevent complications with complex patient discharges or with patients who require lots of medical equipment in the home."[31]

Although home health services at HMC are nurse led, a multidisciplinary team plans and coordinates care to meet individual patient needs. "This approach is a major factor in our success, and our patients and their families appreciate interdisciplinary care delivery," says Scruby.[31] To support this approach, case conferences are held with all members of the multidisciplinary team present, including the home care physicians. Each patient has a unique medical record for home health services in which all members of the multidisciplinary team plan and document the care given to a patient. This process enables all health professionals to access information about a patient and the care being provided by another member of the team. "This is certainly useful when a home care patient is admitted to an inpatient facility and discharge is being planned as it provides background about past care provision and previous health care requirements," says Scruby.[31]

Staff members in home health services also work closely with patients and family members to coordinate care, enabling them to be proactive in meeting the patient's needs in the home. "We communicate with patients and family members closely prior to discharge," says Scruby, "We talk about what's going to happen when the patient is discharged home, how often we will visit, what we can do for them, what to do if there is a problem out of hours, and also discuss any of their fears."[31] Because of the open lines of communication between staff and patients or family members, Scruby notes that patients and family members are very proactive in phoning if there is an issue. Finally, home health staff members assess patients and their caregivers or family members for their education needs. For instance, if patients will be discharged home with oxygen therapy or wound care dressing changes, patients and caregivers will be given specific education in those areas. "A patient educator role has been developed to go out to patients who might need extra education in a particular area," says Scruby. "And our pharmacists will also go out to educate patients on their medications."[31]

Barriers

Even with the improved case management processes and the implementation of the liaison case manager in the hospital, staff in home health services struggle at times to ensure that patients have a smooth transition to home health services. "For example, we cannot perform miracles when we've been given short notice on a complex discharge for a patient requiring lots of medical equipment in the home," says Scruby.[31] In addition, HMC would like to improve the medication reconciliation process for those patients transitioning from the hospital to home health services. New referrals come to home health services with a written referral from the physician along with a list of the patient's medications.

"The clinical pharmacist and physician review the medications on admission, as well as the liaison case manager or a case manager in the home health services," says Scruby. "At times, it can be difficult to assess the medications the patient was taking at home and what he or she will be taking upon discharge from the hospital. We are looking at electronic systems to improve medication reconciliation and make it more simplified."[31]

Results

Overall, the initiation of the liaison case manager role in the hospital has improved patient transitions from receiving care in the hospital to the home. In addition, monitoring whether current patients receiving home health services have been admitted to the hospital helps staff prepare for those patients' eventual discharge back to the home. "To further evaluate our progress in transitioning patients to the community with home health services, we look at patient satisfaction surveys, quality management indicators, and survey results from Joint Commission International," says Scruby.[31]

References

1. Joint Commission Resources: Project RED: A green light for better hospital discharge procedures. *The Joint Commission Benchmark* 12:3–4, Jan.–Feb. 2010.

2. Jack B., et al.: A reengineered hospital discharge program to decrease rehospitalization: A randomized trial. *Ann Intern Med* 150:178–187, Feb. 2009.

3. Society of Hospital Medicine: *The Project BOOST Mentoring Program.* http://www.hospitalmedicine.org/ResourceRoomRedesign/RR_CareTransitions/html_CC/project_boost_background.cfm (accessed Jul. 19, 2010).

4. Mark Williams, e-mail message to Julie Henry, Apr. 1, 2010.

5. Tina Budnitz, telephone interview by Julie Henry, Mar. 29, 2010.

6. Snow V., et al.: Transitions of Care Consensus Policy Statement: American College of Physicians, Society of General Internal Medicine, Society of Hospital Medicine, American Geriatrics Society, American College of Emergency Physicians, and Society for Academic Emergency Medicine. *J Hosp Med* 4:364–370, Jul. 2009.

7. Snow V., et al.: Transitions of Care Consensus Policy Statement: American College of Physicians–Society of General Internal Medicine–Society of Hospital Medicine–American Geriatrics Society–American College of Emergency Physicians–Society of Academic Emergency Medicine. *J Gen Intern Med* 24:971–976, Aug. 2009.

8. Farquhar M., et al.: Barriers to effective communication across the primary/secondary interface: Examples from the ovarian cancer patient journey (a qualitative study). *Eur J Cancer Care* (Engl) 14:359–366, Sep. 2005.

9. Nissen M., et al.: Views of primary care providers on follow-up care of cancer patients. *Fam Med* 39:477–482, Jul.–Aug. 2007.

10. Babington S., et al.: Oncology service correspondence: Do we communicate? *Australas Radiol* 47:50–54, Mar. 2003.

11. Snyder C., et al.: Trends in follow-up and preventive care for colorectal cancer survivors. *J Gen Intern Med* 23:254–259, Mar. 2008.

12. Efrat Shadmi, e-mail message to Julie Henry, Mar. 12, 2010.

13. Kerzman H., Baron-Epel O., Toren O.: What do discharged patients know about their medication? *Patient Educ Couns* 56:276–282, Mar. 2005.

14. Shadmi E., et al.: Cancer care at the hospital-community interface: Perspectives of patients from different cultural and ethnic groups. *Patient Educ Couns* 79:106–111, Apr. 2010.

15. Divya Shroff, e-mail message to Julie Henry, Feb. 26, 2010.

16. Joint Commission Resources: Case study: Creating a safer anticoagulant therapy system through communication. *The Joint Commission Perspectives on Patient Safety* 9:9–11, May 2009.

17. Helen Siegel and Mary Ann Preskul-Ricca, telephone interview by Julie Henry, May 21, 2010.

18. Joan Spicer, telephone interview by Julie Henry, May 26, 2010.

19. Kohn L., Corrigan J., Donaldson M.: *To Err Is Human: Building a Safer Health System.* Washington, DC: Institute of Medicine, 1999.

20. World Health Organization (WHO): *Safe Surgery Saves Lives.* Geneva: WHO, 2009.

21. The Joint Commission: *Meeting The Joint Commission National Patient Safety Goals.* Oak Brook, IL: Joint Commission Resources, 2009.

22. Shojania K., et al.: Making health care safer: A critical analysis of patient safety practices. *Evid Rep Technol Assess* (Summ): 43:i–x, 1–668, 2001.

23. Schiøler T., et al.: Incidence of adverse events in hospitals: A retrospective study of medical records. *Ugeskr Laeger* 163:5370–5378, Sep. 2001.

24. Davis L.: The Danish health system through an American lens. *Health Policy* 59:119–132, Feb. 2002.

25. Strandberg-Larsen M., et al.: *Health Systems in Transition.* Geneva: World Health Organization, 2007.

26. Louise Rabøl, e-mail message to Julie Henry, May 29, 2010.

27. Patient Safety Research Conference: Climbing the Patient Safety Culture Ladder; Hospital Staffs Evaluation of Safety Culture in Hospital Departments; Survey Among 21,123 Staff Members in the Capital Region of Denmark. Porto Portugal, 2007.

28. Lundgaard M., et al.: The Danish patient safety experience: The Act on Patient Safety in the Danish health care system. *Ital J Pub Health* 2:64–68, 2005.

29. Danish Society for Patient Safety: *Handbook of Safe Team Communication.* Hvidovre, Denmark: Danish Society for Patient Safety, 2007.

30. Hamad Medical Corporation: *About Qatar: Health Services.* http://www.hmc.org.qa/hmcnewsite/qatar.aspx#Health_Services (accessed Jul. 5, 2010).

31. Vicki Alexandra Scruby, telephone interview by Meghan Pillow, July 4, 2010.

Index